APPLIED KINESIOLOGY

Shows how the study of muscle movements and their relationship to the rest of the body's complex systems can provide a practical and reliable means of diagnosis and therapy.

APPLIED KINESIOLOGY

Muscle response in diagnosis, therapy and preventive medicine

by

Tom & Carole Valentine

THORSONS

THORSONS PUBLISHING GROUP
Wellingborough · New York

Published in the UK by Thorsons Publishers Ltd., Denington Estate,
Wellingborough, Northamptonshire NN8 2RQ, and in the USA by
Thorsons Publishers Inc., 377 Park Avenue South,
New York, NY 10016.
Thorsons Publishers Inc. are distributed to the trade by
Inner Traditions International Ltd., New York.

First published 1985

British Library Cataloguing in Publication Data

Valentine, Tom
   Applied kinesiology
   1. Kinesiology
   I. Title   II. Valentine, Carole
   III. Hetrick, Douglas P.
   612'.76   QP303

   ISBN 0-7225-1123-X

Printed and bound in Great Britain

Acknowledgements

The authors owe a considerable debt of gratitude to Douglas P. Hetrick, D.C. and David S. Walther, D.C. This book could not have been written without their generous help. Dr Hetrick's professional excellence and continual search for ways to improve his medical art were the initial inspiration for the book. In treating Tom Valentine for several health conditions, he patiently explained procedure after procedure. He also patiently checked the manuscript and corrected errors in anatomical fact. Dr Walther, Diplomate of the International College of Applied Kinesiology, is the founder and publisher of Systems D.C. in Pueblo, Colorado. Information from his textbooks, pamphlets and brochures is an integral part of this book. Not only do the authors owe Dr Walther a debt of gratitude for all his help, but the practice of applied kinesiology owes him its gratitude for his many years of dedicated research, clinical observations and excellent texts.

Contents

Chapter One:

Introducing Applied Kinesiology

In a brief session, a competent applied kinesiologist can evaluate your various bodily functions by testing your muscles, and then present you with a fairly accurate picture of how your glands, organs, lymphatic system, nervous system, circulation, and muscle and bone structures are working.

It's a rather bold claim, but valid, in our experience. Applied kinesiology (AK) is a practical and reliable diagnostic tool and holistic therapeutic modality that has emerged in the past twenty years or so. AK appeared in 1964, and it has grown impressively. Today there are hundreds of competent clinical and practical researchers contributing to the ever-growing body of knowledge. Since the practice was founded by a chiropractor, it makes sense that most applied kinesiologists are chiropractors. However, over the years other physicians, including dentists, M.D.'s, podiatrists (chiropodists), osteopaths, and even psychiatrists, have learned the art. Today we may approach an applied kinesiologist with confidence.

The list of health problems that the applied kinesiologist can address confidently and helpfully is impressive and still growing. For example, children with chronic sniffles or other nagging cold symptoms may benefit from a muscle-testing session. Or, if you are in need of a change in diet to knock off some fat, or merely to improve your energy level and sense of well-being, an AK session will help determine which nutrients you really need before you go to the trouble of breaking old habits and preparing new foods. Maybe you're thinking of jumping on the fitness bandwagon and plan to start running a few miles each day. If so, a muscle-testing session could help you avoid the chronic problems that might develop from faulty structure. Athletes, young and old, amateur or professional, would do well to have their body functions analysed regularly by a competent AK practitioner. These are but a few of the uses to which competent applied kinesiology can be put.

This book is designed to tell you everything you need to know about AK from a patient's point of view. Our resident expert, Douglas Hetrick, D.C., of Escondido, California, has been effectively applying kinesiology in his chiropractic practice for five years, and our guest experts include some of the original geniuses behind this new and exciting healing art form.

The word 'kinesiology' is derived from the Greek and generally translates as 'study of motion.' In this case it refers to the study of the mechanics of bodily motion, especially muscle movements and their relationship to the rest of our complex body systems. 'Applied' means simply 'put to a practical use.' All the physicians who have taken the time and effort to learn about AK have learned to put it to effective use.

A personal example can clearly illustrate how applied kinesiology works on an average person — me. My condition, when I first met with Dr Hetrick to discuss this book, was that I was more than forty pounds overweight. In addition, I am a lousy patient — the kind who does what the physician says only if it isn't too inconvenient. Prior to Dr Hetrick's initial examination I had learned from various other experts that I was probably hypothyroid. That means my thyroid gland, which controls my body metabolism, wasn't doing much of a job. Physicians tell us that glands may be 'hypo' (too little activity) or 'hyper' (too much activity). Obviously my body had not been metabolizing, or burning up fats very well. The standard solution for hypothyroidism is the element iodine. I had already been taking several drops of an expensive iodine solution every day for a year, on the advice of a licensed nutritionist, but it didn't appear to do me any good.

One ten-minute session with Dr Hetrick showed that my thyroid was suspect, but not necessarily because of lack of iodine. (Later we were to learn that it wasn't iodine that my body needed, but something else.) Dr Hetrick tested only two of my muscles in that first brief session, and the way they reacted told him what he needed to know. (This was a brief, first examination; more detailed explanations will follow in the main text of this book.)

After quickly checking my skeletal-muscular balance Dr Hetrick 'tested' my left forearm, which actually gave him information about my shoulder muscle. Having a strong skeptical streak, and having been forewarned about the possibility that 'suggestion' might play a role, I questioned him on what he was about to attempt. He said that a particular muscle in my forearm, the left teres minor, would test 'weak' if my thyroid was not performing properly. He was prepared to prove to me the validity of his testing procedure. He gripped my arm in a certain way, then told me to resist strongly when he pushed it down. Then, to my surprise, as I strained against his pressure, he overcame my resistance with the ease of a circus strongman.

'Now,' he said, 'put your finger here,' and he poked me moderately with his finger at a spot on my upper left pectoral. The spot actually hurt from his moderate pressure. When I placed my own finger on the spot, it was also tender to my touch. That particular spot marked a juncture of lymph and nerves that he said was associated with the thyroid gland. The claim is that finger pressure somehow 'therapy-localizes,' or isolates, the thyroid, and that when the teres minor muscle test is then repeated, the muscle may test 'strong.'

I did resist much more strongly on the second go round! Now my curiosity was aroused. Just touching that spot on my chest seemed to make my arm muscle stronger. Remove the finger and, strain as I might, the muscle was weaker. This, Dr Hetrick explained with a confident grin, could mean that my thyroid gland was malfunctioning. However, he required further diagnosis, especially temperature taking, before he could determine the precise nature of the malfunction.

Dr Hetrick's years of experience suggested to him that there was a likely connection between my thyroid malfunction and another set of glands. He suggested a second test. I was to lie on my back while he checked my right leg. I have always been proud of my leg strength. My legs may not be very long, but they are miniature tree trunks. 'Resist,' the physician commanded when he was in position, cradling my leg so that I could resist with only one or two particular muscles, and not an entire set. I resisted, and this time I tested 'strong'.

Feeling smug, I eagerly awaited the next test. This time he had me place the fingers of my right hand on my abdomen, on the right side about midway between diaphragm and hip. With my finger firmly in place on another spot, I resisted again. This time my strong leg muscle tested decidedly weak. Surprised at this, I demanded, 'Do that again, Doc.' This time I gritted my teeth and psyched up my strength for the test. He tested me again, and I was weak! However, when I removed my finger from the spot, which he said related to the adrenal glands, I could practically lift him off the floor.

That brief encounter told the physician that my adrenal glands were somehow misfiring, and there was probably a relationship between that malfunction and my thyroid problem. I didn't need to donate a gallon of blood or urine for testing in a laboratory. Nor did I require overnight hospitalization in order to take a BMR (basal metabolic rate) first thing in the morning — a test, incidentally, that usually shakes up the testee so badly that the results are tarnished.

How accurate was this mini diagnosis? How did the follow-up exams and subsequent therapy work? Would this work for you? That's what this book is all about.

Doug Hetrick was not our first encounter with applied kinesiology, but his years of experience and his considerable patience in explaining the complex theories behind the practice certainly made him the most thorough. Years ago I heard about the new practice that was sweeping through chiropractic, especially in the Midwest, where I lived and worked as a reporter. Applied kinesiology was then not yet a decade old, but already it was struggling with image problems. This is invariably the case in the healing arts — anything new is always viewed with considerable suspicion and resistance. The founder of AK is George J. Goodheart, a Detroit chiropractor, and the resident genius behind the International College of Applied Kinesiology (ICAK), the authorized training body for the practice. In 1973 there was no ICAK, and some overzealous, would-be healers attended a seminar by Dr Goodheart and emerged with self-proclaimed 'miracle' healing ability. This sort of behaviour did not help the credibility of early applied kinesiology. One exuberant Chicago-area practitioner, evidently fresh out of college pre-med classes, muscle-tested an acquaintance of ours, and informed her that her tubes were blocked and she could never have children. He also diagnosed her as a cancer victim. Sensibly, she balked. A second opinion found that she was already pregnant and had no signs of cancer. The last word we had on the deviant kinesiologist was that he had decided on a return to medical school.

That kind of blatant quackery, which occurs in every professional healing field, delivered a severe blow to AK, and even today one hears derogatory remarks about it from both the medical establishment and various uninformed gossips. A primary aim of this book — and of the entire *Inside Health* series — is to tear away the veils of misinformation and provide a more balanced view.

Bear in mind that the most prestigious medical doctor at the most prestigious medical facility, following the most prestigious and expensive set of diagnostic and exploratory evaluations, including surgery, is still pretty much guessing, and is dependent upon his years of practical experience, when he attempts to discern a cause of bodily misfunction. This is especially true in cases of chronic and metabolic ailments as opposed to clear-cut germ pathologies. You and I know this about medicine, and yet we place a great deal of faith in our orthodox medical doctors — and rightly so! The wonders of modern medicine are impressive. If I suffered from a heart problem, for example, I'd not hesitate to trust any number of today's qualified heart specialists.

Our position in this entire series of books is not an adverse position; rather it is an adjunct position. Applied kinesiologists demonstrate that they are capable of testing the body with the body. This has definite advantages. They use a whole, walking, talking person, as opposed to testing one who is anesthetized or drugged and probably desperately sick. The differences between standard diagnostics and AK's muscle testing is staggering when you compare expense and human suffering. There is no way that AK can replace much of today's crisis medicine, but that is not its purpose. Applied kinesiologists are far more interested in health than in disease. Their goal is to prevent serious illness, thereby taking some of the heavy load off the shoulders of our overcrowded hospitals. An open and fair comparison of the claims of AK with those of 'establishment' medicine should demonstrate that applied kinesiology deserves ample equal opportunity to prove itself. Thus far the opportunity has not been equal, but the applied kinesiologists have made the best of it.

Applied kinesiologists look at every person from a 'triad of health' perspective. This is the three-sided nature of every human being that makes up a healing art's triangle of *structure, chemistry, and mentality.'* We discuss this extensively in Chapter 2. At this point we shall just point out that chiropractors approach health and healing from a 'structural' basis, medical doctors generally from a 'chemical' basis, and psychiatrists and psychologists from a 'mental' or 'emotional' basis. Most applied kinesiologists, being 'holistic physicians', attempt to work with all three areas of health, and in some cases they include a 'spiritual' dimension. Doug Hetrick stresses the holistic approach, as do an ever-growing number of physicians today.

Applied kinesiology originated in 1964 when Dr Goodheart encountered some puzzling muscle behaviour. He noticed that a particular patient exhibited a weak serratus anticus muscle on one side. The serratus anticus muscles are designed to hold the scapula the ('wing-bone' behind the shoulder) to the ribcage. If one of these two muscles is stronger than the other, it can pull the shoulder out of kilter, causing all kinds of problems. Dr Goodheart was puzzled because the weaker muscle did not seem to be atrophied, or withered. He examined the muscle with his fingers and found some painful nodules (little bumps) where the muscle originates at the ribs (see Figure 1).

Curious to learn whether these nodules were affecting the strength of his patient's wing muscle, Dr Goodheart deeply massaged the nodules, then retested. He observed that the muscle

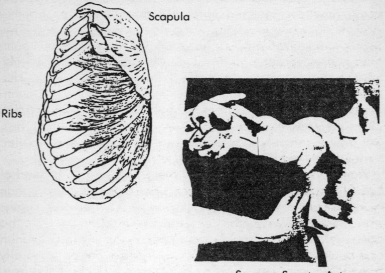

Scapula

Ribs

Squeeze Serratus Anticus

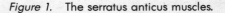

Figure 1. The serratus anticus muscles.

has gained considerable strength. Thus was born a technique for muscle therapy called 'origin-insertion,' which was the precursor of applied kinesiology.

The origin or head of a muscle is its starting point, the fixed attachment that serves as the basis for muscular action. In contrast is the muscle's *insertion,* the point where the muscle is attached to a more moveable part. When a muscle contracts, in order to exert force, the action demands that the insertion always move towards the origin. This is why the AK doctor is so specific when preparing to test one of your muscles. It's not magic; it's knowing the exact direction of muscle movement.

Further experiments with the patient led Dr Goodheart to observe specific relationships between muscle weaknesses and other physical conditions. Dr Goodheart's early work was valid enough to interest other chiropractors in learning manual muscle-testing procedures for diagnosing conditions pertaining to structural balance. Muscle testing is one way an AK chiropractor can find the precise location along your spine where something is out of place. Another method is X-ray. Correlating the two methods was one way early AK diagnostics were confirmed.

From those humble origins, applied kinesiology blossomed into a major diagnostic art as more and more qualified practitioners and researchers entered the field.

Our complex body systems provide five avenues of diagnostics and/or therapy to the applied kinesiologist. These five bodily avenues are: (1) the nervous system, (2) the lymphatic system, (3) the vascular (blood vessel) system, (4) the cerebrospinal fluid, and (5) the meridian system (that is, the acupuncture lines). The fifth system is taken directly from the ancient healing art of acupuncture, which came to public attention in the United States at about the same time AK was getting off the ground. Dr Hetrick stresses that all five systems are so intricately interwoven, each with the other, that it is impossible to separate them. To the applied kinesiologist the body functions as an integrated whole, and must be tested as such. AK therefore stresses that the whole is, indeed, greater than the sum of its parts. It is thus able to make sense of vague complaints of the 'I just don't feel well' variety.

This last point may have a profound effect on medical thinking. It may even demolish the lopsided statistics dealing with hypochondriacs — those people who allegedly 'imagine' their sickness when nothing is physically wrong. A medical doctor once told me that nearly 80 per cent of his patients were 'hypochondriacs' who had 'nothing wrong with them at all.' In light of what applied kinesiologists have learned, a diagnosis of 'hypochondria' may prove to be an excuse for ignorance or insufficient diagnosis on the part of the physician. Establishment medicine requires that the patient present a specific disease or clear-cut symptom in order for the physician to treat the problem. Because of this specialization it is difficult for doctors to deal with vague descriptions of general malady. Thus, despite its many triumphs over disease, modern medicine has often been baffled in the face of various chronic and metabolic ailments.

This is where applied kinesiology may be of assistance. The

purpose of *Applied Kinesiology* is to inform you of the potential applications of AK for you and your family, to describe how it works, and to explain how you can be assured of competence when you seek a practicing AK physician.

Chapter Two

The Triangle of Health:
Structure, Chemistry, Mentality

The term 'holistic' has emerged from relative obscurity in the 1960s to play a leading role in alternative medicine and in the social awareness of health. 'Holistic' derives from the philosophical term 'holism', the theory that 'whole entities, as fundamental components of reality, have an existence other than as the mere sum of their parts.'

The applied kinesiologist is a holistic practitioner par excellence.

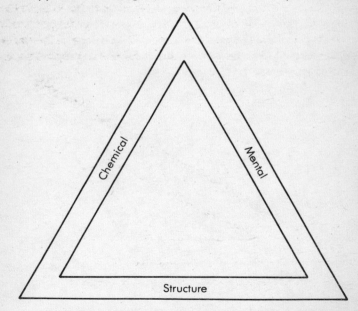

Figure 2. The triad of health.

He (or she) deals with the interrelated whole of your body and personality, and utilizes those interrelationships in his diagnostic technique.

David S. Walther, D.C., a diplomate of the International College of Applied Kinesiology, wrote the definitive textbook of AK. The first volume, *Basic Procedures and Muscle Testing*, opens with an in-depth discussion of the triad of health. The triad includes structural, chemical, and mental sides of the human being, as indicated in the equilateral triangle in Figure 2.

Chiropractic, which gave birth to AK, is based upon the structural side of human nature. This does not mean that chiropractors ignore the other two sides of our nature; it simply illustrates the emphasis of their practice. Doug Hetrick explains that 'the competent AK cannot be lopsided in his practice and effectively treat his patients. He must deal with every person holistically as an equilateral composite of the triangle.'

You and I might assume this view to be so basic as to be taken for granted by all medical practitioners, but such is not generally the case. Medical doctors generally specialize in one of the three, thereby enlarging the triangular framework out of proportion, as shown in Figure 3.

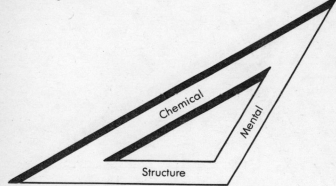

Figure 3. Imbalance in the triad of health.

The general practitioner automatically prescribes drugs, or chemicals, for pain and other symptoms. Usually the patient gets rapid relief from the symptom even though the cause of his illness may be structural or mental. Indeed, the essential appeal of chemical treatment — and the resulting wealth and power of the pharmaceutical industry — came about precisely because drugs do alleviate painful symptoms quickly. Unfortunately, in many cases they also allow the patient to neglect the underlying problem and prevent the body from healing itself.

Philosophically there should be very little conflict between medical specialities, especially if the holistic approach is generally accepted. Conflicts of opinion, however, are generally based on economics rather than philosophy, although the latter is always held up to the light of controversy. No physician will admit, 'I prefer my method because it makes me more money.'

Regardless of what you hear, or read, your health is determined by your whole being, and in the *Inside Health* series we treat every aspect of medicine and health as fairly as possible.

The idea of specializing is certainly not wrong, although it has led to general controversy and some instances of over-specialization. Figure 4 illustrates the triad of health as observed

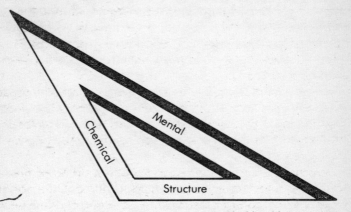

Figure 4.   Imbalance in the triad of health.

from the psychological point of view. Most psychiatrists, psychologists, psychotherapists, hypnotherapists, and other counselors of mental and emotional disorders approach your whole being from that necessarily lopsided point of view.

Dr Walther drew Figure 5 to depict how chiropractors, podiatrists, orthopedists, rolfers, physical therapists, dentists, naprapaths, and osteopaths generally view the triad.

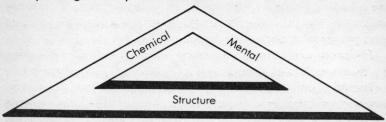

Figure 5.   Imbalance in the triad of health.

Surgery is based in structure, and the leading cause of medical necessity continues to be direct physical trauma — injury to some part of the body. When the body is broken, bruised, and busted, the therapeutic approach of the structurally oriented physician is outstanding. The surgeon repairs the damage, or the chiropractor corrects the subluxations or spinal misalignments, and the body can then heal itself. Who has not been touched by awe when learning that surgeons managed to sew an arm or hand back onto a victim of accidental amputation, restoring the limb to normal or near-normal use?

Unfortunately, as Dr Walther points out, 'many times the patient's chief complaint — a structural problem — originated on another side of the triad. This is when the structurally oriented professional obtains no improvement, or gets improvement only to have the condition return.'

Now we are entering the second greatest arena of medical concern after direct trauma — the chronic ailment, the nagging aches and pains that signify something is wrong or going wrong.

Dr Hetrick, observing my complaints of pain in the lower back, neck, and feet, as well as sundry 'charley horse' muscle aches, pointed out: 'Some structural stress might be due to a primary chemical or mental stress — this has become common knowledge — so all my structural approaches will be either unsuccessful or temporary until the chemical-nutritional or mental stress is eliminated.'

It is interesting to note that AK practitioners almost always qualify 'chemical' with the term 'nutritional.' The reason the word 'nutrition' generates particular interest here is that we live in a world of marketing and advertising media wherein drugs or chemical potions are glorified out of proportion to reality. In fact, the single greatest 'chemistry' in our bodies is nutrition. To live is to eat, to be nourished, and all nutrients are essentially chemical.

Coincidentally, my personal complaints matched the text of Dr Walther's classic example. 'There are many mechanisms by which mental and chemical stress can affect body structure,' he writes. 'A classic example is functional hypoadrenia (poorly performing adrenal glands), which in turn affects the sartorius and/or gracilis muscle strength. These muscles are very important anterior stabilizers of the pelvis; when weak, they allow structural strain to develop.' Dr Hetrick and other AK doctors see a great deal of this type of malady — the chronic back or neck pains caused by terrible nutrition. Until I began work on the *Inside Health* series, I was addicted to several cups of strong coffee a day with cream and honey or sugar. Carole finally goaded me out of the habit. Few bad habits can overstimulate the adrenals and wear them down as caffeine in coffee does.

Yes, that first cup of coffee gave me a 'lift' every morning. It 'whipped' my adrenals for me. I needed a second lift shortly after, and another after that because of the inevitable pendulum swing we cannot escape in nature. What goes up must come down. My overworked adrenals were on a roller-coaster ride, and it didn't take long for my body chemistry to be loused up. Weary and worn adrenals affected my sartorious — the long muscle that starts at the front of the pelvis (anterior superior iliac) and runs down to connect with the front part of the inner knee (tibia). The sartorius flexes the knee and hip, rotates the thigh laterally, gives support to the knee, and in reverse supports and flexes the pelvis on the hip.

For years I had complained of back pain. A smart pain served as my morning alarm clock for nearly thirty years, arousing me promptly at six daily regardless of the firmness of my mattress.

I learned to live with it and continued my coffee and other bad dietary habits. When I finally sought a chiropractor, the back pain had entrenched itself moderately all the way up from the coccyx (tailbone) to the base of my neck. The chiropractor pushed and pulled and clicked my spine, and the sharp pains subsided shortly thereafter. The dull pains remained, but I was happy.

Periodically my back would 'go out', and I would return for manipulation. Many people lose patience with their physicians because they must continue returning for treatment. Such returns are economically sound for the physician and the economy at large, but not for the individual. I began seeing a chiropractor for the first time at the age of thirty-five. More than a dozen years later, I have experienced the handiwork of several chiropractors from various schools, naprapaths (who concentrate on musculature rather than spinal alignment), massage therapists, and other structural practitioners.

'My structural corrections will be ineffective like all the rest,' Dr Hetrick explained, 'unless you correct the nutritional deficiencies causing the problem.' Nutrition has long been ignored by orthodox allopathic medicine, but that ignorance is slowly being corrected as the philosophy of holism is being reborn. The diagnostic practice of applied kinesiology may soon lead the way as it steadily overcomes entrenched skepticism.

Dr Hetrick has encountered cases that illustrate the interplay among the sides of the triad given in Dr Walther's textbook:

One woman's chief complaint was headaches, but she also had digestive problems manifested by gas and heartburn. She was embarrassed by the digestive symptoms and reluctant to talk about them. She turned out to be a textbook example of a structural trauma affecting the person's body chemistry. This interplay is why my evaluation of a patient's condition is so lengthy and detailed.

This particular patient had sprained an ankle more than a year ago. She assumed it had healed and the problem was gone forever. However, she decided to go jogging with her husband regularly, and the subluxations of the foot and ankle caused by the severe sprain earlier improperly stimulated the proprioceptors whenever she was standing, walking or running. [Proprioceptors, found throughout tissue of the muscles, joints, and tendons, respond to stimuli and emit nerve impulses or messages.] The improper proprioception caused structural stress in the suboccipital area [lower back of the head] and this inhibited other muscular action while she jogged.

The patient experienced mild headache in the suboccipital region, but these vanished with a good night's sleep. Eventually the wrong messages caused cranial faults that interfered with normal vagus nerve activity. This in turn reduced the secretion of hydrochloric acid, which affected the production of pancreatic enzymes, and naturally led to poor digestion.

The added stress of her chronic headaches further aggravated her condition — it was literally a vicious circle.

Later we shall deal with proprioceptors and the vicious circle of structural disorders affecting chemical affecting mental affecting structural *ad infinitum*. The point of this case is clear. The only solution to the patient's headache and indigestion problems lay in finding and correcting the ultimate cause. Muscle testing, the essence of applied kinesiology, and careful questioning finally determined the true source of the problem, and it was corrected. Not instantly, but over time with proper treatment.

Treatment with aspirin and antacids had done nothing to cure the woman's problem, though it may have dealt with the painful symptoms. However, since her hydrochloric acid was deficient, the antacids were causing more digestive damage in the long run.

'Doctors specializing in only one side of the triad,' Dr Hetrick said, 'can generally give only partial results, if that. My chiropractic adjustments to the patient's cranial and upper back brought only partial and temporary relief until the foot and ankle cause was isolated, and repaired.'

Even the best of natural nutrition, along with supplemental hydrochloric acid and digestive enzymes, would have remedied only part of the problem.

The added stress of dealing with chronic headache could have sent the patient to a psychiatrist, but without a dynamic evaluation from applied kinesiology, the basic foot-ankle problem would continue undetected.

My own case, lower back pain, matched the classic textbook case of chemistry affecting structure — the direct opposite of the case cited by Dr Hetrick. In today's society both examples are extremely common. Active people sustain minor trauma that is ignored or 'heals' quickly but results in improper proprioception. Or 'normal' people eat a lot of junk food and over time suffer from malabsorption and perhaps mucous congestion in the small intestine. The small intestine is associated with the abdominal muscles and the quadriceps (front upper thigh from knee to hip), and these muscles are vital to the stabilization of the pelvis. When weakened, they allow the pelvis to rotate toward the front, increasing the lordotic (backward-bending) curve of the lower spine and jamming the 'facet articulations,' which is technical language for parts of the vertebra. This makes your abdominal muscles so weak you can't do situps without twisting to call upon the strength of other muscles.

In 1975 I suffered a severe stomach ulcer problem. It was eliminated by, of all things, acupuncture after liquid antacids and other chemicals failed miserably.

The point is made. I was among the millions who evidently sustained structural stress (and pain) from a basis in faulty nutrition or, more properly, faulty nutritional chemistry.

Examples of chemical factors affecting mental factors also abound. The major symptom is depression. The same faulty nutritional chemistry can affect the glandular secretions and cause a syndrome leading toward hypoglycemia. 'Syndrome' is a term for a series of vague rather than specific symptoms, and 'hypoglycemia' means low blood sugar.

An example of the mental affecting the chemical may be menopausal symptoms of hot flashes and severe fatigue. It is known that emotional stress has a powerful effect upon the adrenal glands. In the classic case, the wife of an alcoholic is the victim of tremendous daily stress. All treatment of her chemical and structural symptoms will fail until the emotional trauma caused by her husband's drinking is eliminated.

'Sometimes a patient does not want to talk about deeply personal problems, so the physician does not know they exist. In applied kinesiology we can continue to monitor certain signs given in muscle testing that tell us to question for emotional trauma,' Hetrick explained.

There are also probabilities of the mental affecting the structural. Dr Walther gives the example of the wife of an alcoholic under duress coming up with symptoms of colitis. While being treated for the colitis with a bland diet, the woman develops lower back and leg pain. Chronic colitis will cause a weakness in the tensor facia lata muscle (front of hip to outer knee) somehow activated by the neurolymphatic reflex that affects both the colon and the muscle. When this muscle weakens, a subluxation around the second or third lumber is probable, and presto, back pain.

The reverse is also possible — structure affecting mentality. Dr Walther cites 'rolfing,' as described by Ida Rolf, as an example of a physical therapy being used to overcome psychological problems. In the textbook case, an auto accident victim sustained a structural impairment to the pelvis. This disorganized proprioceptive communication to the rest of the body. The end result, following a complicated route through the body systems, was schizophrenia. Dr Walthers writes: 'There is always a causative factor; it remains to be found for correction of the condition. In this case, the chemical and structural sides of the triad must be corrected to eliminate the mental factor.'

Dr Hetrick points out that in his experience, and in that of other AK practitioners, it is extremely rare for a chronic condition not to feature, to some extent, involvement of all three sides of the triad. What person can sustain a physical injury without some mental stress and chemical reaction in the body?

The challenge of the applied kinesiologist is to find the primary involvement so that the basic cause of the ailment may be determined. Of course the secondary conditions may also require therapy, but the component AK physician wants to end the patient's need for treatment by treating him or her holistically.

A thorough AK muscle-testing program is also an excellent way to catch symptoms or syndromes in the early stages of development. This is one reason AK is in the vanguard of the modern movement of preventive medicine.

Chapter Three:

What Applied Kinesiology Can Do For Your Family

Used properly, applied kinesiology can help you and your family over any number of potential health problems.

Suppose you have a chronic malady, meaning that it persists, or comes and goes more or less regularly, despite various forms of treatment. A common example might be the syndrome of symptoms that has come to be known as the 'common cold.' If the symptoms of the common cold recur in you every other month for a few days, you might do very well to visit a competent applied kinesiologist. No doubt all the chemicals in the drug industry's bag of tricks have already been tried with only a modicum of success.

As we pointed out earlier, AK is the only branch of the healing arts that appears to be fully equipped to deal with the general malaise — the 'I just don't feel good' syndrome. Perhaps you or a family member have a glandular malfunction that isn't critical enough to display 'serious' symptoms yet. Your body is perhaps a year or so away from needing to be rushed to a hospital. The general malaise is your body's way of telling you that something is amiss — one of your sparkplug wires is misfiring, perhaps. Unlike an automobile engine, your body has far more than four or six cylinders to run on, so the misfiring is compensated for. Yet something just isn't right, and you don't feel well. AK muscle-testing procedures can detect the essence or beginnings of a problem before it becomes acute, with obvious symptoms.

Medical doctors prescribe remedies for specific symptoms, but are generally powerless to deal with general malaise, except, perhaps, to say, 'Take two of these pills and call me in the morning.'

It is not the fault of the physician, it is a shortcoming in the nature of their training. Often an M.D. will consider a patient complaining of general malaise to be hypochondriac, or a person who only 'imagines' he is feeling poorly. Applied kinesiologists strive to avoid such helplessness when faced with a lack of obvious symptoms.

In the words of Dr Goodheart, 'Applied kinesiology is based on the fact that the body language never lies. The opportunity for understanding the body language is enhanced by the ability to use muscles as indicators of body language.'

Dr Goodheart is not claiming miracles; he claims that AK physicians may enhance the ability to interpret the body's signals as relayed by the muscles.

Dr Goodheart continues: 'Once muscle weakness has been ascertained, a variety of therapeutic options is available. The opportunity to use the body as an instrument of laboratory analysis is unparalleled in modern therapeutics because the response of the body is unerring; if one approaches the problem correctly, making the proper and adequate diagnosis and treatment, the response is adequate and satisfactory both to the doctor and to the patient.

Applied kinesiology, therefore, is not a 'magic bullet,' which is medical jargon for a miracle cure that is not yet in the industry's bag of tricks. However, a competent AK practitioner may, indeed, perform vital health services unmatched in the healing arts.

Imagine, if you will, all the common chronic complaints tormenting the population: back pain, headaches, asthma, cold syndrome, allergies, slow recovery from bumps and bruises or breaks and sprains.

Carole is fond of saying that health begins with motherhood and the developing child, assuming of course, sound genetics. So, to illustrate the value of AK diagnostics for everyone, we begin at the beginning — pregnancy.

Doug Hetrick, always the chiropractor with his emphasis on structure, nodded in agreement when we suggested that mothers-to-be were ideal candidates for an AK diagnostic examination series. 'Every pregnant woman,' he said, 'would profit from applied kinesiology. There are many possible problems areas that not only may affect the mother, but might affect the developing child as well.'

One of the most common potentials, which AK is particularly adept at discovering, is the condition I experienced — hypoadrenia. 'If a mother has this glandular problem,' Dr Hetrick remarked, 'the developing child's adrenals will try to supplant the shortages and, in turn, also become hypoadrenic.' Dr Walther has explained that hypoadrenia in a developing baby often leads to allergies.

Functional hypoadrenia, incidentally, is a perfect example of a developing health problem that is not acutely symptomatic. If your adrenals fail, you have Addison's disease, and that's another matter entirely. Applied kinesiology helps the physician diagnose the adrenals' shortchanging problems long before the malicious symptoms occur.

Dr Walther also pointed out that in the late period of the pregnancy the mother's body secretes a hormone called relaxin, which instructs the pelvic ligaments to soften so that the baby can be delivered. During this particular secretion period muscle imbalances may easily cause spinal and pelvic problems that later become chronic back pain or headache.

After the child is born and is busy growing, good pediatric care should include AK muscle testing and evaluation. Structural imbalances in the muscles and bones of a growing child can lead to chronic pain in maturity.

The holistic approach has shown that our bodies are a wondrous complex of nerve and energy patterns that operate the living entity. It's important here to recall the five systems of the 'intervertebral foramen' mentioned earlier: the nervous system, the lymphatic system, the vascular system, the cerebrospinal fluid, and the meridian system.

Chiropractic proved long ago that spinal imbalance and dysfunction can cause interference with normal nerve function, which, in turn, causes misfunction in organs and glands. AK telescoped the interworkings of the various systems further still, and today it is observed in AK that the various muscles of the body are on particular nerve and energy patterns, which can be correlated with particular organs and their functions. If a particular muscle is weak, the deficiency may be in any one of the associated energy systems, indicating a possible deficiency in associated organs or glands.

Additionally, chiropractors have known for a long time that when a muscle is weak, a deviation occurs in the structure it supports. A person who habitually holds his head tilted to one side, for example generally has a weak neck muscle on the opposite side. It's usually that simple.

Growing children may be watched closely by parents, with occasional help from an AK practitioner, and potential problems may be detected in the child long before any symptomatic malady occurs. Generally the imbalance you observe at such an early stage

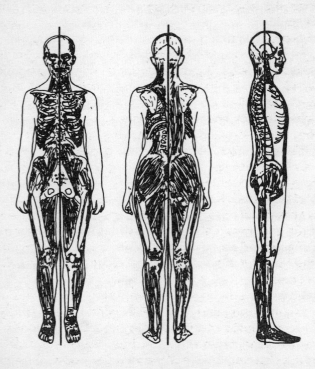

Figure 6.   Observing structural balance.

is easily corrected. Dr Walther has produced a small handout brochure to help parents evaluate their child's structural balance. It states:

> It is especially important to consider structural balance at the time of athletic injuries, jarring falls while playing, or at the onset of complaints such as headaches, backaches, leg aches, fatigue, asthmatic wheezing, or other ailment. There are no such things as 'growing pains'. These pains are real. They are the result of improper body function which causes pain to notify the body that something is wrong. Normal growth is not a painful process.

The brochure then explains that the best way to observe structural balance is with a plumb line (a string with a weight on one end, hanging in a straight line from ceiling to floor), as shown in the drawings in Figure 6.

Dr Walther advises that you check your child's posture when he or she has little or no clothing on. What you are looking for when viewing both the front and back as aligned along the plumb line is symmetry. The two sides of the body should be symmetrical, evenly distributed.

Observing from the back, Dr. Walther writes:

> The head should be level, not tilting to one side or the other. This can be observed with the plumb line or by observing the height of the ears, which should be level.
>
> The shoulders should be level. Check this by sighting across the shoulders or observing the length of the two arms. The hands should be rotated the same amount on each side, and the palms should face slightly backward. The elbows are slightly bent in a relaxed position, not straight or excessively bent.
>
> The shoulder blades should be of equal height and equal distance from the midline. They should be solidly against the back chest wall and not 'flared out.'
>
> The spine should be straight, with a balanced elevation of the musculature on each side.

The waist is normally curved on both sides, not having a straighter appearance on one side.

The hips should be of equal height. A good way to observe this is to find the bony top of the hip with your hand. Place one hand on each side; observe whether your hands are level.

The gluteus maximus [buttocks] should be equally rounded on both sides.

The legs should be basically straight, showing no knock-knees or bowleg appearance. Sighting along the Achilles tendon (back of heel), you should see a straight line down the leg to the foot, with no roll-over of the foot in either direction.

Next, you check the front of the child's body. The brochure goes on:

Have your child open and close his mouth. His jaw should swing straight down and not deviate to the right or left.

The shoulders should not roll forward excessively, nor have a hollow appearance just medial to the shoulder (between the neck and the end of the shoulder).

The chest should be equally developed from right to left.

The legs should not rotate to either side or to the center. You can best see this by looking at a kneecap and observing that it is directed straight forward. If there is rotation, there will be greater space from the edge of the knee to the edge of the kneecap on either the medial or lateral side.

The feet should point slightly outward and to the same degree on both sides.

When you check the side view of your child's body, Dr Walther suggests you pay particular attention to the ankle, knee, pelvis, shoulder, neck and ear.

Observe for excessive forward curve of the neck or forward position of the head. The upper mid-back region frequently has an excessive backward curve.

Observe for a sway-back condition in the lower back.

The pelvis can sometimes tilt forward or back as a total unit.

The knee should not have an excessive forward or backward position in reference to the plumb bob.

Observe for overall rotational factors in your child when his feet are side by side. There should be no rotation of the pelvis, shoulders or head.

Any of the imbalances you are looking for may signify a weak muscle, which may signify a weakening pattern along one or more of the five diagnostic avenues outlined in Chapter 1, which, in turn, might uncover nutritional deficiencies, or some minor injury never brought to your attention — or any number of signals about the child's potential health.

Parents who are interested in the holistic approach would do well to visit an accomplished AK practitioner periodically and consult with him directly on the best way to observe for structural balance.

The brochure closes with a brief discussion of watching your child in motion for clues to structural imbalance. The key, once again, is balance between the two sides of the body. Watch for tendencies to throw one leg, or roll a foot inward, or run with one arm swinging more than the other.

When I was a youngster the idea of good posture was primarily cosmetic. 'Stand up straight, young man!' was heard often and my mother also criticized girls of my age who 'hunched over' and didn't stand erect. Applied kinesiology delves far deeper than good appearance when a postural evaluation of a child is made.

Imagine an adolescent boy or girl with poor posture being constantly nagged and belittled for deliberately slouching, when in fact the poor posture is due to a weak muscle condition, or an inadequate diet. The resulting stress problems are left to your imagination. Dr Walther states:

Good function is balance between the two sides. Many times poor balance and poor structural integrity are classified as 'awkward' or 'clumsy.' This awkward or clumsy appearance is often present when a child cannot function efficiently because of disturbances to certain energy patterns within the body.

When an imbalance is observed — whether it be postural slouch, clumsiness, or whatever — nagging the child to change will rarely improve the condition. It is impossible for a child to remember all the time what good posture is when his body is assuming an imbalanced position because of improper muscle strength.

Consistent postural problems are rarely the result of laziness. Muscular imbalance from poor nerve supply or other energy patterns literally will not allow the child to stand erect. He needs help, and you can give it to him. Examination and treatment by a physician knowledgeable in applied kinesiology should be done early.

Thus, throughout growth and maturation, a holistic approach spearheaded by AK analyses makes very good sense.

A physical examination by an M.D. will be enhanced by an AK analysis. In fact, Dr Walther, in his instructions to AK physicians, insists that AK be used in conjunction with standard diagnostic and evaluation techniques.

Chapter Four:

Your First Kinesiology Examination

Have you ever felt apprehensive and a little intimidated in the face of a physical examination at a hospital or doctor's office? If you have, you'll be relieved to know that your experience at the applied kinesiologist's provides a gentle contrast.

First, you are not necessarily ill when you go for an AK exam. You are making the visit to *prevent* malady. You will be examined, but you will not be pricked with a needle, probed with stainless-steel instruments, or filled with some chalky liquid to facilitate X-rays.

'In applied kinesiology,' Dr Hetrick explains 'we start on the surface, and like most physicians we strive to treat the obvious. However, our goal is to uncover the basic underlying cause, and AK techniques are designed to challenge and test and treat, then challenge and evaluate again until we've covered all the possibilities. We've learned that this is the only way to obtain permanent correction of a problem.'

The AK evaluation is not the variety of 'preventive maintenance' that standard medical examinations have offered for decades. Standard preventive health care traditionally means visiting your doctor every year or so for blood and urine tests and a general physical. Such periodic checkups are fine, but consider this: in order for something to show in your standard evaluational procedures, a disease of some type must already be manifest! 'The ideal,' Dr Hetrick points out, 'is to discover causative factors before they've been around long enough to cause an actual pathology.'

This does not mean that the applied kinesiologist does not value the various diagnostic tools available to modern medicine. The competent AK physician makes the appropriate referrals, often discovering a serious potential health danger long before standard procedures might do so. For example, Dr Hetrick has on several occasions encountered telltale muscle-testing reactions that indicated a potential for heart problems and immediately recommended the patient to visit a cardiologist for a complete check-up.

The obvious question that arises here is, did the AK muscle testing prove correct? Were the heart recommendations valid? Generally speaking, yes. However, the AK procedure may indicate a potential heart condition before any overt symptoms are available for the cardiologist to find. One of the inherent values of AK muscle testing, or the reading of body language, is that it does not depend upon symptoms that the patient can describe. Body language betrays dysfunction before symptomatic patterns are formed.

At your first AK examination, be prepared to have your body language tell on you. At the time I was undergoing AK treatment, I had been working to overcome my weakness for coffee. After a few months of sessions with Dr Hetrick, I deliberately enjoyed two cups of coffee, before visiting him, with plenty of cream and sugar.

'What did you do?' He asked in amazement as he tested the leg muscle that indicated adrenal function. I was impressed. He didn't know precisely what I'd done, but he certainly knew I'd done something. I chalked up another score for applied kinesiology, then confessed. Prior to that day I had been totally off coffee for two months.

So be prepared, and, for heaven's sake, don't lie about the junk food you eat if you want the physician to help. Researchers around the world know how much people lie about their diets. Kidding yourself and your doctor will only slow the AK evaluation down.

Your body speaks to the knowledgeable AK physician. Dr Walther, in his definitive textbook, writes:

The language of the body — and understanding it — can be likened to a page of Chinese script. Most of us in the western world would ignore it because we couldn't understand it. To someone who knows Chinese, it might be a most valuable document. As more information about body language is decoded, subtleties such as movements, structural distortions, colors, etc., have a great value in determining why health is not at an optimum level. The doctor who learns applied kinesiology progressively asks more often, 'Why is that?' rather than simply accepting that the unusual motion, response, or color is something different in this patient.

In the previous chapter we talked about postural evaluation for children. Well, nothing's changed. Now your structural balance is going to be evaluated. And the practiced eye of an AK physician will see much more than the gross distortions.

Generally, we pass each other daily without paying any attention to forearm rotation, shoulder level, or head tilt in one another. The tailor making a fine suit of clothes notices differences like these and covers them nicely. When we do notice that someone's eyes, for example, are not exactly the same size or shape or level position, we may shrug it off with the old saying 'Nobody's perfect.' It even seems that slightly mismatched eyes must be 'normal.' But are they?

According to AK principles, our bodies *should* be essentially in balance. Dr Walther writes, 'One often fails to observe important body language factors simply because the factor is thought to be a normal variant within the population. To become aware of these structural changes, always remember that *nothing* takes place within the body without a reason' (emphasis added). He goes on to say that noticeable differences are not usually due to right- or left-handedness, nor to congenital anomalies.

'Learning to read body language properly is like anything else,' Dr Hetrick notes. 'You have to study and practice and educate yourself.' In many cases with physicians, understanding body language is a matter of re-education, or perhaps 'undoctrination.' For example, in his text Dr Walther stresses that most physicians are taught during college that the cranium is a fixed structure, that there is no movement in the skull. Not so! 'Study of the skull *in vivo* [alive and kicking as opposed to a dead skeleton] reveals apparent definite movement,' writes Dr Walther.

Admitting that the term 'apparent definite' smacks of jargon, let's hear Dr Walther out: '. . . there is evidence of interference with a person's health if that movement [of the living cranium] is not proper. Indications of a cranial fault can be observed by a symmetry of the skull and facial muscles. These are difficult to observe until the significance is realized.'

It is not our purpose to educate you in the AK profession, but knowing what the AK is supposed to know will help you understand why you are paying that professional in hard-earned currency.

In his textbook, Dr Walther included the following about the AK physician's skill in interpreting body language:

Ability to observe variants requires systematic study of subtle, frequently imperceptible, qualities. The author is reminded of the first time he observed Goodheart 'reading body language.' Here was an individual standing behind a patient he had never seen before, making observations about the patient's spinal structure, abnormal function, points of strain and general health characteristics in more detail than most doctors could after a thorough examination. This knowledge about the patient was developed from visual observation only; it was found to be highly accurate after discussion with the patient and the actual examination. Many of the observations were made from a mere shadow caused by a slightly bulging muscle on one side, which was not apparent on the other side. The reason Goodheart was able to determine the patient's symptoms prior to discussion or examination was his highly developed ability to see muscular imbalance, and to tie that knowledge together with his knowledge of muscle-organ association.

Finally, the competent AK physician is trained in understanding the various energy patterns within the body. From the ancient tradition of acupuncture, AK physicians have learned the meridian system's value in diagnostics. It has been discovered that when there is an energy imbalance within the meridian system, the body will reveal this information by thermal variances at different areas of the skin.

Sometimes a sensitive instrument called a thermocouple is used to measure these variances in temperature; at other times the apparent heat differences are evaluated subjectively by the physician. You may experience coolness in a specific part of your body, yet the physician or his equipment may fail to confirm the temperature difference. AK has methods for testing the particular meridian that coincides with that 'cold spot' and for further evaluating the organ structures associated with that meridian. Chances are your 'feeling' regarding that cold spot is correctly identifying a deficiency — a deficiency en route to becoming a symptom, perhaps.

The AK examination is likely to refresh your memory of various little aches and pains that come and go. It's virtually impossible for a patient to remember everything experienced by the body, and most minor complaints vanish shortly after making their presence felt. Pain sensed at alarm points along specific meridians generally gives the AK physician information about particular muscles and organs. This information leads him to ask questions during the examination that may help you recall body facts lost to memory.

'Well, I did sprain my ankle about a month ago, but it was nothing. It's healed now,' a person might say. Or 'I hit my head on the shower nozzle, but the bump is gone now.' Or 'Well, I do get sleepy after eating a big meal, but isn't that normal?'

Incidentally, the phenomenon of 'referred pain' is not new, nor particularly special with AK. Many forms of referred pain are recognized generally. For instance, pain in the shoulder and arm may occur with heart problems, and pain in the second thoracic vertebra (upper back) may be associated with a gallbladder attack.

Although the AK physician recognizes the value of meridian therapy (acupuncture or acupressure treatments), he is taught that meridian activity is merely the indicator and seldom the culprit. In instances where the meridian is the culprit, however, acupuncture becomes an amazingly effective modality.

After the AK physician observes all your little imbalances, he will continue the examination with various 'challenges.' This means he is going to generate some kind of stimulation to the wondrous complex of energy patterns, muscle, bones, circulation, and other elements that make up your body, and see what reaction occurs.

This is the beginning of AK's speciality — muscle testing. This is where the 'smart-alecky' patient can try as he might to fool the indicators, only to have the competent physician show him up at once. That last observation comes from the voice of experience.

In the profession, it is understood that with specific challenges, all muscles of the body will temporarily be less able than usual to resist a specific testing procedure. In other words, even if there's nothing wrong, the AK physician can tamper with a stress point or meridian or whatever and reveal a 'weakness' in the particular muscle.

Therein lies a potential for chicanery, which we will discuss later.

The challenges may be either positive or negative. A positive challenge can be made by asking you to place your fingertips at a certain point. You may recall that when my thyroid-associated muscle was tested, and tested weak, Dr Hetrick had me place my finger on my pectoral muscle at a particular, slightly sore spot, and my own touch apparently strengthened the reaction.

Challenges may also come in the form of nutritional factors. Dr Hetrick gave me a particular nutritional compound. He placed a tablet in my mouth, and naturally my salivary system went to work. The thyroid-associated muscle tested weak, which indicated to him that this was not the proper substance required. A different supplement tablet was placed in my mouth, and this time the muscle tested strong, indicating that my body had a use for the particular nutrient.

There is controversy here. Nutritional allergy-testing procedures by AK physicians are under fire from the medical establishment — a subject dealt with later.

'Adjustments' may also be part of the AK examination. In chiropractic, spinal manipulations seem to vary considerably from one practitioner to the next. A chiropractor of slight build, treating a large patient, might literally jump on the patient to adjust him. Snap, crackle, pop go the vertebrae, and the patient is either better or in worse shape. Today many chiropractors are of the opinion that the snap-crackle-pop school is of little or no value. The subluxations and fixations of the spine that are causing problems may be adjusted and corrected without all that crackling.

The AK physician will make an adjustment — with or without the crackling, which often cannot be helped — and immediately follow with a specific muscle test to see if he's done the job properly.

During the examination procedure, challenges with various structural manipulations may be commonplace.

All three sides of the triad of health — structure, chemistry, and mentality — will be used during the examination's challenge sessions. If a psychological trauma is associated with a particular problem, your muscle will test accordingly when the AK physician suggests you think about the traumatic matter. This doesn't sound so much like hocus-pocus when you consider that the standard lie detector records instantaneous physiological reactions to mental or emotional events.

The challenges help the expert read your body language, and the various challenges of particular muscles through the triad will help him to eventually ferret out the cause of what ails you.

When Dr Hetrick had me place my fingers on my pectoral muscle, he was engaged in what is called 'therapy localization.' The phenomenon that occurs when the patient touches an area on his own body that is not functioning was first noticed by Goodheart years ago. Admittedly, more research is required before the mystery of why this technique works is fully revealed, but as the eminent medieval philosopher Roger Bacon once wrote, 'Man can do more than he knows.' The AK physician can accurately diagnose with the process of therapy localization, even though he has only theory to explain his results. Continual double-checking with other forms of diagnosis and treatment over the decades has built up a strong confidence in the body of AK knowledge.

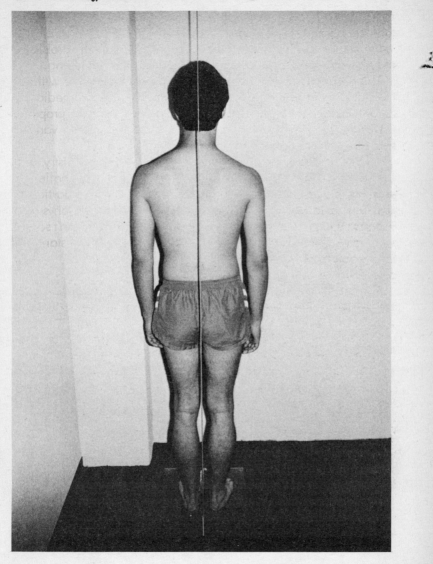

Photo 1. Examination begins with a plumb line analysis. Sam's right shoulder is low, his right ear and right hip are high. He's not in balance.

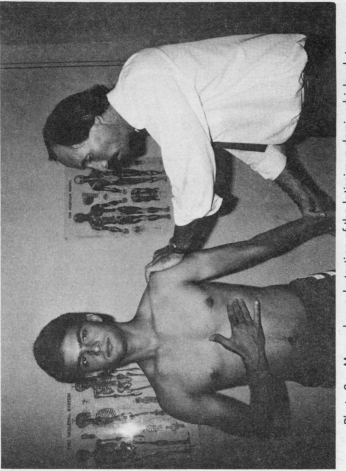

Photo 2. Manual muscle-testing of the latissimus dorsi, which relates to the pancreas. Sam's right middle fingers are therapy-localizing the neurolymphatic point associated with the pancreas.

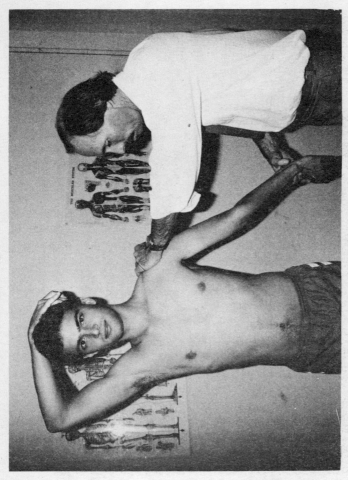

Photo 3. Manual muscle-testing of the latissimus dorsi, continued. Sam's right hand over his head to his left temporal region (note his fingers) is therapy localization of neuro-vascular association with the pancreas.

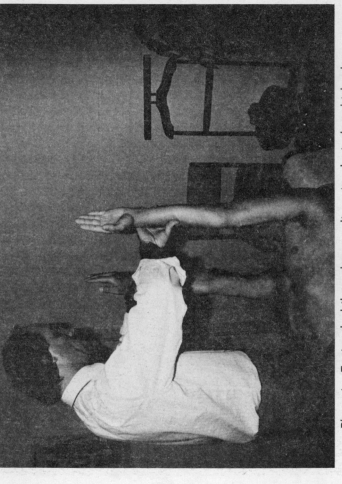

Photo 4. Testing the bilateral pectoralis major clavicular which relates to the temporal bulge, cranial fault, potential and possible hypochlorhydria (not enough stomach acid). Dr Hetrick will pull the arms apart as Sam resists.

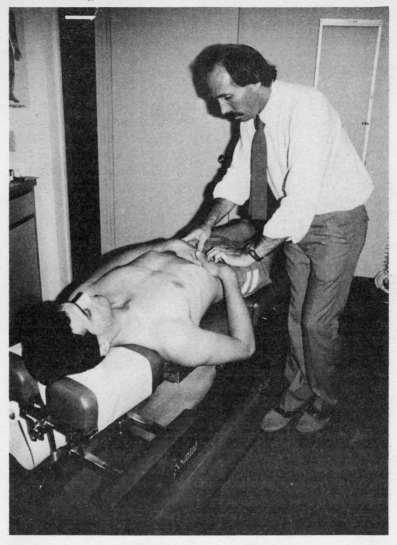

Photo 5. Dr Hetrick helps Sam place his hand at his ileocecal valve. The ileocecal not closing properly is a common 'just don't feel good' syndrome cause — the patient may feel disoriented, nauseous, have a bad taste in mouth, etc.

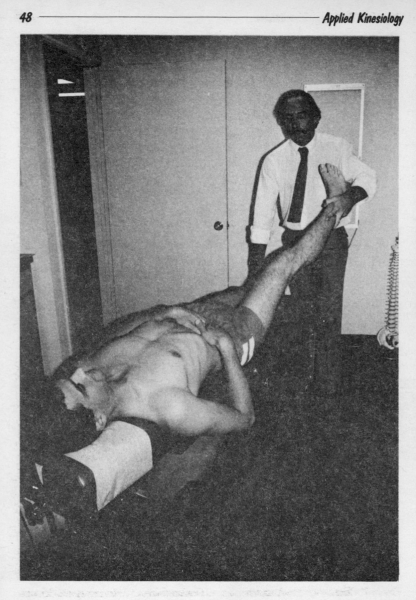

Photo 6. Manual muscle-testing the tensor fascia lata muscle related to the ileocecal valve.

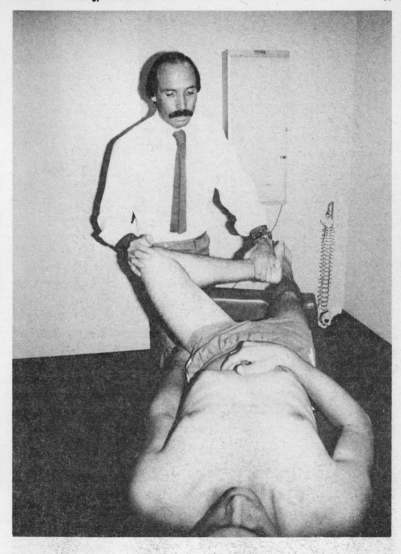

Photo 7. Testing the left sartorius, which is related to the adrenal. Sam's right fingers touch the neurolymphatic point associated with the adrenals to therapy-localize during the diagnostic procedure.

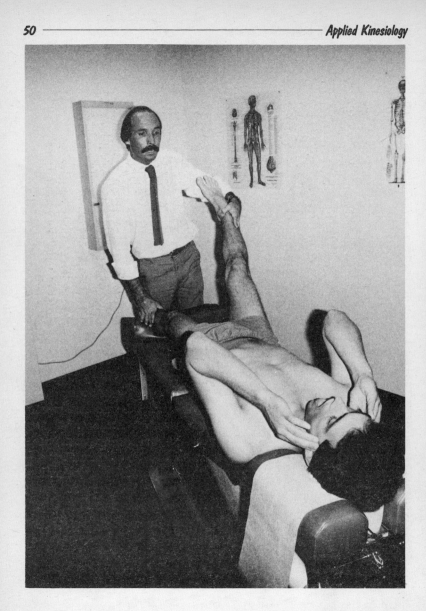

Photo 8.   This time the therapy localization centers at the jaw joints as
Dr Hetrick tests the tensor fascia lata muscle.

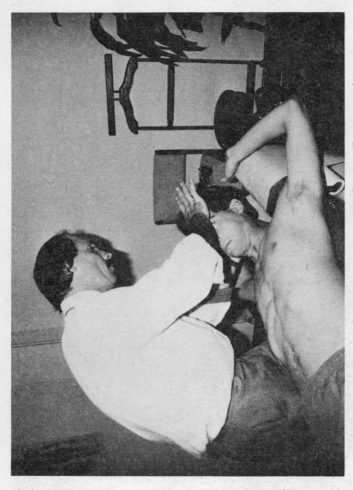

Photo 9. Manual muscle-testing the neck flexors. These muscles are related to the sinuses, and also inform the physician about neck and head imbalances.

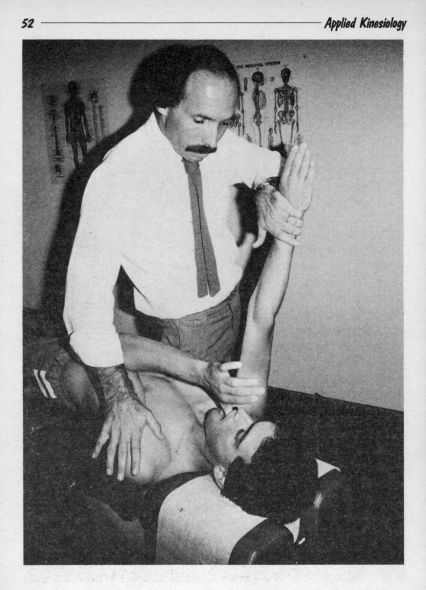

Photo 10. Sam's thumb presses against his palate to therapy-localize for a spheno-basilar cranial fault as Dr Hetrick tests his pectoralis major clavicular.

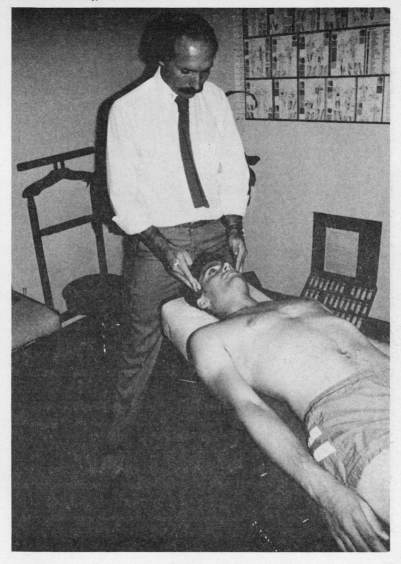

Photo 11.   This is not a manual muscle test. This is a palpation of the temporal sphenoidal line.

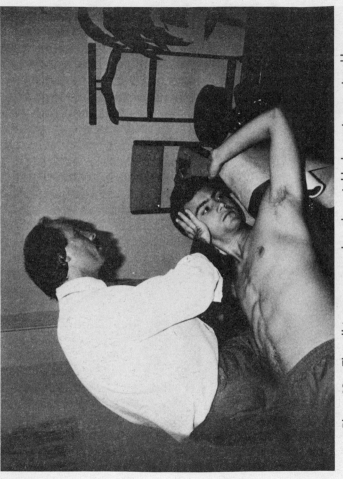

Photo 12. The all-important neck and cranial balance is examined by testing the sternocleidomastoids (SCMs). Here Dr Hetrick tests Sam's right SCM.

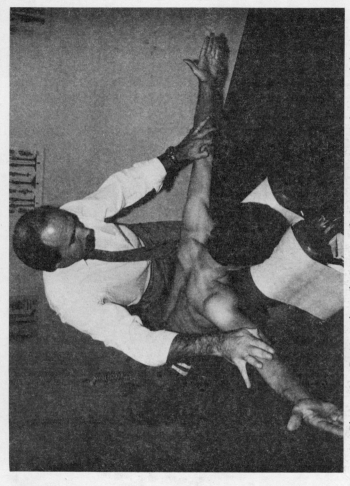

Photo 13. Dr Hetrick is about to push Sam's arms straight toward the floor as he resists. This is testing the bilateral lower trapezius muscles. If they test weak it may indicate a fixation in the dorso-lumbar region of the spine.

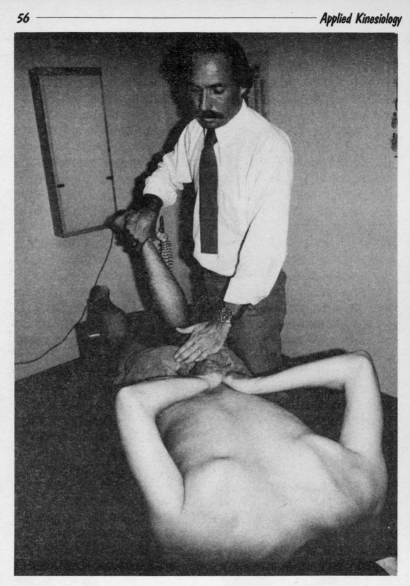

Photo 14. Both of Sam's hands are used to therapy-localize while Dr Hetrick tests his hamstring. The association is with muscles in the pelvis and with proper orientation of the pelvic girdle.

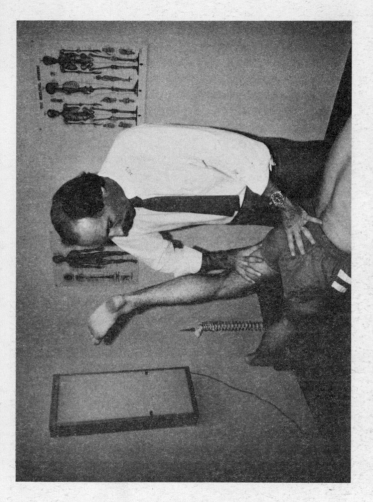

Photo 15. The gluteus maximus test is related to the reproductive system and to pelvic balance.

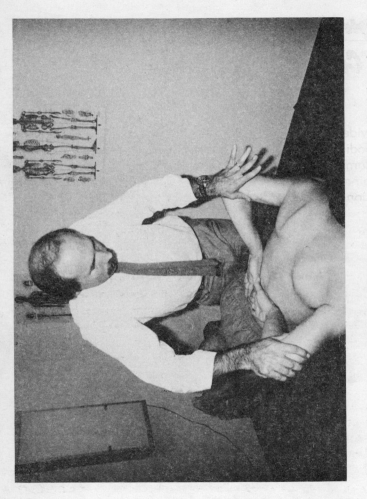

Photo 16. Again downward pressure will be applied to test the bilateral teres major muscles, which are related to thoracic fixations.

Chapter Five:

Checking Your Glands and Organs

It is widely accepted today that environmental stress wears down our bodies every day in a number of ways, and many of us have the damnable knack of making things worse for ourselves. The combined stresses of pollution, poor nutrition, overindulgence, emotional trauma, and just living in the rat race help make medicine in general the third largest revenue-producing field of endeavor after agriculture and manufacturing.

The AK physician knows how the stress of everyday living takes its toll, especially on our adrenals. He also knows, from years of experience, which nutrients might best replenish which types of glandular or organ depletion he encounters in a patient. The AK muscle-testing procedures, when concentrated upon nutritional and chemical factors, reveal the state of our glands and organs — much to the benefit of our future health.

Testing the chemical side of the triad of health while the patient is up and around, so to speak, has tremendous advantages. After all, you are walking, talking, and breathing normally while your system is being evaluated. That certainly beats waiting until you've got to be anesthetized and cut open so that a surgeon can peer inside and say, 'Yes, it's a mess!'

Chemical technology is one of the wonders of our modern world. The cynic might retort that it's a wonder we've survived it this long. Chemical weed killers and insecticide bathe much of our produce; chemical preservatives keep food products on the shelves longer and make them more economical, but not necessarily more digestible. Chemical exhausts spew forth into the air and other pollutants enter water, fog, and rain.

Being able to test our physiological reactions to chemistry — which includes nutrition, the most vital chemistry of all — is, to many, the most exciting aspect of the AK art. In his textbook, Dr Walther opens the subject cautiously and thoroughly, as follows:

The body's reaction to chemicals, including nutrition and adverse chemicals, can be tested by manual muscle testing. This influence will be revealed by a muscle strengthening or weakening, depending upon the compound being tested. Upon administration of the compound, there is an immediate influence on the muscle function. This suggests that the influence is by way of the nervous system. The neurologic pathways that influence muscle strength — either positive or negative — are *speculative* [emphasis added]. It is obvious there is brain activity as soon as a substance is chewed; we immediately know whether we like the substance or not. This, of course, is from the stimulation of the nerve endings dealing with taste. It is possible that the central nervous system, recognizing the compound being ingested, relays information to the organs and glands, preparing for use of the compound. If the compound is recognized as beneficial, the energy pattern is immediately enhanced, influencing not only the organ or gland, but also the associated muscle.

The term 'energy pattern' is used often by AK physicians and it has various levels of meaning. The familiar lines of force one can see by placing a magnet beneath a paper sprinkled with iron filings provide a commonly observed 'energy pattern' or the pattern of the magnetic field. Electromagnetism is a pervasive force in the physical universe and every element in the atomic table resonates, or vibrates in harmony, with electromagnetic energy in a distinct manner. In simplistic terms, a particle of carbon will inscribe a particular pattern when jolted by a specific electrical charge, and a particle of calcium, or one of iron, will inscribe its own particular pattern when charged by an identical jolt. Energy emanates from chemical compounds and is absorbed by chemical compounds in wavelengths or frequencies. Every cell in an organism resonates with specific frequencies of energy. In addition to this aspect of cellular energy, the 'energy pattern' would also include fields surrounding areas of energy activity. In this regard, energy patterns of the organism would include the negative and positive nature of electrical charges. All these aspects are loosely lumped together when the term 'energy pattern' is discussed by AK physicians. Additionally, the term can describe a broader phenomenon: for example, the patterns drawn around the body by the acupuncturist are invisible, but can be demonstrated by both the acupuncturist and the AK physician.

Dr Walther and many other researchers are theorizing that the body's reaction to chemicals ingested is determined by a complex series of actions and reactions involving the energy patterns of the substances ingested and the body cells. 'Our bodies might be affected by food energy patterns of which we are not currently aware.' To test one aspect of this thesis, Dr Walther conducted an experiment wherein certain foods were subjected to the high-intensity energy of a microwave oven. He determined that the irradiated foods sustained a distorted 'food energy pattern.' This was proved by muscle-testing patients after they ingested foods that had been irradiated in the microwave, and conducting the same muscle testing after the patients ate the same foods, but unirradiated.

'The irradiated material was effective only occasionally, but nutritional products which had not been irridiated were effective as would usually be expected,' he said. In other words, muscles tested weak with irridiation most of the time and strong without it, as anticipated.

Dr Walther stressed that his test was 'double-blind' — that is, neither the doctor nor the patient knew which food product was test or control material. He suggests that continued testing be performed in this manner so that statistical data can be obtained to further evaluate his hypothesis.

Whether or not Dr Walther's experiment proves anything about energy patterns inherent in food, the evidence that the microwave somehow affected the nutritional value of foods adversely supports contentions by many researchers that microwave cooking may not be optimally healthful.

Incidentally, Dr Walther was quick to point out that his experiment was not conclusive because of the considerable number of variables involved. Every individual is biochemically unique.

AK practitioners have learned from experience just how varied and unique each individual can be. Coffee, for example, does not affect every person the same way, and people will show different body language reactions to refined sugar, another good example.

You may raise a skeptical eyebrow at the notion that the nutritional effects on the body of something ingested can be tested by the strength or weakness of particular muscles, but consider this: Nerve impulses travel at about the speed of light, or the speed of electronic circuitry, and our blood circulates faster than the speed of sound. Suppose a curare-poisoned dart were to strike someone in the neck. How much time would pass before the victim became paralyzed? Not very long at all — experts tell us it is only a matter of seconds. So, if the body recognizes nutrients and other chemicals instantly — and we can certainly discern flavors in the twinkling of an eye — it seems reasonable that the integrated energy systems of the body will react to these substances instantly. That's the theory, in a nutshell.

That the body recognizes and reacts instantly to nutrients and other chemicals is difficult to refute. Dr Walther suggests that chewing our food, for example, serves purposes other than those known at this time. We know that breaking up food with our teeth and mixing it with saliva helps start the process of digestion. But there may be still other physiological activities vital to digestion that are stimulated by chewing food. 'This seems obvious,' Dr Walther writes, 'since skipping this stage of ingesting food is detrimental to an individual.' He gives the example of children who have severely damaged their esophagi by swallowing caustic materials. Such children are fed ground-up food through an artificial opening cut into the stomach. Even though the ground-up food is balanced and nutritious, the children do poorly. Dr Walther then describes an experiment involving children whose esophagi were destroyed, but whose mouths were intact. They were instructed to chew the food thoroughly, and then spit the bolus out so that it could be placed in the stomach through the artificial opening. 'These children made a remarkable recovery in their total health picture,' he reports.

The correct AK protocol for testing chemical compounds, therefore, is to place the substance in the patient's mouth, on his tongue, so that he tastes the material and the normal chemical reactions of ingestion take place. The physician then tests the associated muscle-organ pattern to determine where there is strength or weakness. It isn't necessary for the patient to swallow the substance for a change in strength or weakness to be identified.

In my case, which involved thyroid and adrenal gland dysfunction, Dr Hetrick tested a number of nutritional compounds in tablet form and found only a couple that my body language agreed that I required. Following a few procedures, you, the patient, can tell how the muscle is reacting just as quickly, if not more quickly, than the doctor can by the feel of your own muscle strength or weakness.

The competent practitioner uses therapy localization to isolate the essence or the cause of a bodily malfunction. My own glandular example is a good one. The examination revealed to Dr Hetrick that I was hypothyroid. Therapy localization, however, showed him that another gland in the endocrine system was the prime culprit, and we soon found my coffee-logged adrenal. How did my body language tell the physician that the adrenal, and not necessarily the thyroid, required attention?

He had me place my finger on the upper left pectoral muscle, which is a thyroid reflex area — meaning that the muscle, gland, nerves and acupuncture meridian involved all mesh within the same energy pattern. When I chewed the tablet of glandular extract of thyroid, if this were the proper nutrient for my condition, the leg muscle being tested would test strong, even though my finger on the pectoral neutralized the pattern or 'localized' the therapy. In this case the muscle didn't test as expected, so Dr Hetrick duplicated the procedure using other substances until one of them strengthened the muscle, indicating it was the substance required.

Time and time again, it has been proved by applied kinesiology that body language does not lie.

AK muscle-testing procedures have been used to prove the adverse effect of certain chemicals on human health. For example, AK physicians have shown that carbon tetrachloride invariably weakens the pectoralis major, which is associated with the liver; or that alcohol will weaken the sartorius and gracilis muscles in

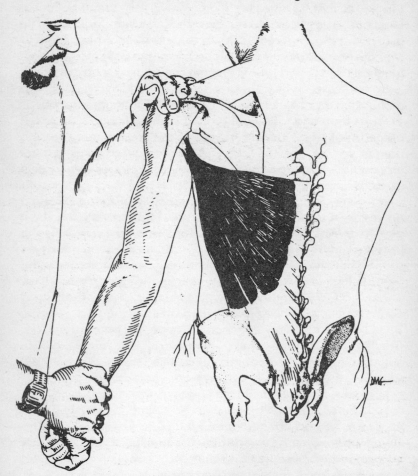

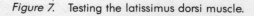

Figure 7. Testing the latissimus dorsi muscle.

an individual with relative hypoadrenia. Since it has been established with certainty that carbon tetrachloride harms the liver and individuals with hypoadrenia suffer particularly adverse effects from alcohol, the muscle-testing indicators generally correspond to what is known.

A common practice among AK physicians, with potential for misuse, is muscle testing for the adverse effects of refined sugar — a dietary no-go in natural-food circles. Because biochemical body conditions are in a constant state of change, this is not an infallible test, but most of the time placing refined sugar on the tongue of a person who is potentially diabetic or has high blood levels of insulin (a cause of hypoglycemia, or low blood sugar) will cause the latissimus dorsi muscle to test weak (see Figure 7). However, a person in a hypoglycemic state at the time of the test would test strong, because the sugar would send signals temporarily strengthening the patterns affected, including the latissimus dorsi, thereby masking the hypoglycemia. Casual or amateurish muscle testing of refined sugar, such as may be observed at various natural food and holistic health expositions are unwise at best.

In addition to taste response reactions, the AK techniques can also test reactions to substances that we breathe in. Researchers have learned that heavy metals, for example, are more readily absorbed by the body when they are inhaled than when they are ingested. One AK researcher experimented with homeopathic compounds and Bach flower remedies by having a subject inhale specially prepared vapors, then testing the muscle responses.

According to Dr Walther, the results in specific conditions, such as upper respiratory involvements or thymus dysfunction, were positive and beneficial to the patient. Since many types of remedies and nutritional factors may be administered and absorbed by inhalation, patients who have trouble absorbing through the gut may be helped.

Chemical muscle testing is most helpful in determining the precise nutrition required by the individual patient. Each of us is biologically unique and we each have our own specific needs — a point driven home by the research of Dr Roger Williams and by that of Dr William Donald Kelley, the maverick cancer researcher who cataloged individual metabolic types.

Dr Hetrick, who attends numerous AK training seminars each year to keep up with new developments in the field, spends a great deal of time learning about human nutrition. 'Standard chiropractic deals with nutrition on a much larger scale than standard medical schools, and AK schooling delves into it in extreme detail,' he says. 'We have learned what traditional healers and housewives knew long ago, that everything taken in by the body has an effect on its health.'

Without individual muscle testing, many nutritional supplements may be a total waste of time or even harmful for certain individuals. 'We have learned that there is a difference in nutritional compounds as they are manufactured by different companies,' Hetrick adds. 'Even though the labels read the same, there are often significant differences which are detected by the individual body.'

Variations in processing and in sources of base materials easily account for these differences. In agricultural science it is well known that the same plants will have varied nutritional value depending upon the soils producing them. This fact has not been stressed to the general public, however, and most people think a carrot is a carrot is a carrot. Dr Walther writes, 'The variance among products and the individual requirements of patients are excellent reasons for testing nutritional products in the patient's own laboratory — his body.'

He also points out that the individual differences that exist in a healthy state are further magnified when health problems occur.

Applied kinesiologists are taught that there are two basic approaches to nutrition. One of them is allopathic, meaning that nutrients are used like drugs. This occurs in megavitamin therapy, which uses massive doses of a particular vitamin or other supplement to correct a specific condition. Some schools of holistic health reject this allopathic approach, arguing that we should heal our underlying health problems by changing our dietary and other habits, not merely by dosing ourselves with concentrated nutrients. On the other hand, crisis medicine certainly has its place, and megavitamin therapy, the subject of another book in the *Inside Health* series, has shown considerable positive results.

Of course, any time the allopathic approach is used, there is the potential for 'side effects.' This is true with megavitamin approaches as well as in drug therapy. 'Massive doses of vitamins, like prescription drugs, are actually an effort to affect a change in body function. The physician is trying to control the body rather than let it do something naturally. This can lead to complications, or side effects,' Dr Hetrick explains.

AK muscle testing has often demonstrated the marked inferiority of synthetic to natural products. The orthodox chemist is taught that there is no difference between a group of molecules put together in the laboratory and those put together by nature. Natural food advocates have long argued that a key difference does exist and that synthetic products lack the living qualities of organic substances. The differences may be extremely subtle, but evidently the body can tell. Dr Walther puts it this way: 'Synthetic vitamins in pure crystalline form are concentrated and use the body's co-factors. This creates the possibility of depleting the body of these necessary items, creating an actual deficiency where none was present. In addition, if certain synergistic elements are not also present, the synthetic vitamin is rarely of any value. Megavitamin dosages of synthetic products can create vitamin toxicity, as is well known with the fat soluble vitamins.'

In addition to synthetic vitamins, the modern diet is generously laced with synthetic substances added to processed foods to refine, preserve, thicken, color, and flavor them. 'It is increasingly evident,' Dr Walther writes,

that in working with nutrition and analysis of the modern-day diet, the refining and concentrating of food products causes *major health problems* [emphasis added]. The concentration of wheat products into white flour and the elimination of the total carbohydrate, which includes indigestible cellulose, are significant problems to the bowel, as there is not enough 'roughage' for a carrier medium. Cellulose is a synergistic material to the refined carbohydrate, even though it may only be one of a mechanical nature. Refined crystalline sugar has lost the synergists that help metabolize the sugar, such as the B complex of vitamins. There is a union of the vitamin B complex and carbohydrate in natural foods. The processing and refining of these foods has divided away the synergistic material necessary to metabolize the carbohydrate. High ingestion of this refined carbohydrate (excessively common today) creates a deficiency of the vitamin B complex. In natural food products, there is an automatic increase of vitamin B complex ingestion when carbohydrates are increased.

AK researchers have learnt that in many cases all of the body's muscles weaken when a high-potency synthetic vitamin supplement is chewed. Muscle testing is therefore used to help determine whether a nutritional substance, either a food or a supplement, may be harmful to a particular patient. An example, from the textbook, is determining whether potassium poses a problem for a patient with my condition, relative hypoadrenia. In this condition it is not unusual for the body to retain an excess of potassium. To verify this, the sartorius muscle (the long one up the inner leg to the front of the pelvis, which is associated with the adrenals) is tested after the patient drinks some potassium-rich unsweetened orange juice. My sartorius tested weak, indicating the juice wasn't doing me any good while I remained in the hypoadrenic state.

Through manual muscle testing the physician can determine with accuracy your body's specific nutritional requirements. Although the correct dosage cannot be determined, the proper substances can be. In some cases the AK physician will determine whether it is best for you to take natural, low-potency concentrations or to take the allopathic approach.

Along with vitamin and mineral supplements, the use of extracts from animal glands and organs — taken by mouth or by injection — has grown as more and more positive results are obtained by health practitioners. Admittedly it is legitimate to question the quality of the materials used for these supplements. For example, would you want to use a calf liver or adrenal extract if the animal was shot through with steroids and antibiotics.?

There are three types of glandular materials used for supplementation in the United States, including whole glandular concentrates, nucleoprotein extracts, and tissue extracts containing hormone substances. A forthcoming book in this series, *Nutritional Supplements,* will discuss the manufacture, processing, and quality control involved in the making and selling of these supplements.

While acknowledging that more research is needed, AK physicians are using glandulars empirically, evidently with good results. Instead of iodine for my hypothyroidism, the manual muscle testing indicated that I'd do better with adrenal extracts. Even though I was a poor patient, seldom doing the exercises prescribed and often sneaking foods not prescribed, after a few months my hypoadrenia appeared to be whipped. My lower back pain of thirty years' duration vanished, and stayed away with the evident strengthening of my right sartorius. Bear in mind, however, that testimonials such as this one are considered highly unscientific. My freedom from pain may be unscientific, but it sure feels good.

Chapter Six:

Testing Your Bones and Muscles

Did you know that the number-one medical problem across the United States, and probably around the world, is plain old backache? According to statistics from the Health Insurance Association of America, more work hours are lost, more pain and misery suffered, and more dollars spent trying to solve back problems than any other single malady.

Applied kinesiology brings new insights into the art of spinal manipulation — the old push-pull, click-click. It is now possible for the manipulator to determine whether his manipulations are worthwhile, at the instant he makes the adjustment. With manual muscle-testing procedures he can 'see' things happening (or not happening) with the vertebra that X-rays would miss.

From top to bottom — from atlas to coccyx — the spinal column is a veritable wonder of bone, muscle, fiber, and fluid. The massive complex of bioelectronic circuitry that automatically operates all our body systems is centered here. No wonder a totally separate branch of the healing arts is centered here as well.

Figure 8 gives you a clear picture of a spinal column. Each part is labeled, in case you're ever a quiz-show guest.

The problems that can occur if any of those vertebral parts gets a little out of line or balance are legion. Our spines are remarkably tough, flexible, and strong, but we find many ways to misuse them and create havoc for our own health.

As is readily observed from my own experience, one does not necessarily need to bend over and pick up heavy objects improperly to suffer chronic back pain. The muscles of the spinal column come in matched pairs, and if one of the pair is weakened

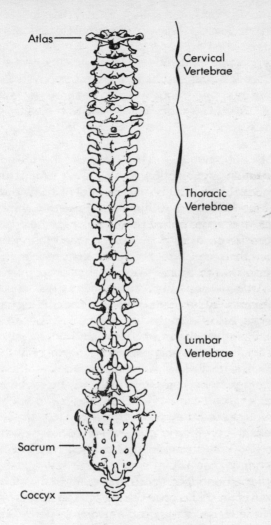

Atlas ——

Cervical
Vertebrae

Thoracic
Vertebrae

Lumbar
Vertebrae

Sacrum ——

Coccyx ——

Figure 8.   The spinal column.

for any reason, the strong one is likely to pull the vertebra out
of optimum position.

Now, there are any number of back specialists who will

manipulate or otherwise place your vertebrae back into proper position. However, if the weakened muscle condition persists, the placement won't hold.

Applied kinesiology offers to back practitioners, especially the various schools of chiropractic, the opportunity to diagnose basic causes of primary spinal muscle weakness or imbalance. AK manual muscle testing also makes the manipulations of chiropractic and other back therapies testable for reliability on the spot.

A back out of whack, in the jargon of the specialist, is either a subluxation or a fixation. Many spine experts use the terms interchangeably, but Dr Hetrick and most AKs differentiate between the two as follows. A subluxation generally involves a single vertebra, or a single portion of the pelvis or the base of the skull, out of precise position. A fixation, on the other hand, generally involves more than one structure because it entails a locking together of two or more vertebral structures.

The AK physician must know that while apparent muscle weaknesses may be associated with specific subluxations, they are not necessarily consistent or reproducible from patient to patient. Therefore the physician should not expect arbitrarily to test indicators for specific subluxations, but must take special notice of individual differences. Fixations, however, feature specific bilateral muscle weaknesses which may be tested in all cases as indicators.

You don't necessarily need to know all this, but your AK doctor had better. The generic problem of backache associates with imbalances, which manifest as subluxations, fixations, or pelvic dysfunction.

When you bend over in the shower to wash your feet and your back 'goes out,' you can generally be sure that the bending over was not the cause of the problem. The spine is designed for all that activity, so the cause is nearly always elsewhere.

'A patient with a chronic upper cervical subluxation,' Dr Hetrick explains, 'probably suffers from suboccipital headaches, which he or she masks with aspirin. The upper cervical problem will weaken almost any indicator muscle in the body when the head is turned or tilted into a particular position. Many times a person will turn or tilt his head into that particular position while bending over, and will therefore experience the back 'slipping out.'

One fellow patient I met at Dr Hetrick's clinic, named Peggy, wrote a testimonial letter regarding her chronic lower back and left leg pain. It was a sciatic condition that had been treated improperly until she had muscle testing. She wrote:

> For three years I sought help from two orthopedic doctors, who could offer me no treatment other than prescribing drugs. To avoid taking drugs, I sought further help by going to a neurologist. He felt I would eventually need back surgery. My experiences left me totally confused. Each doctor came up with a different diagnosis.
>
> Finally, I decided to try chiropractic care. Even though the treatments helped me considerably, the pain would return shortly after an adjustment was made. I became more and more depressed. I lacked energy and had difficulty in gaining weight.
>
> Eighteen months ago I met Dr Hetrick through a mutual friend. His application of kinesiology developed into amazing results. It helped me so much, I feel like a new person. I have renewed energy, the pain I felt in my lower back is non existent, and through his nutritional guidance, my weight is back to normal.

That's a nice letter. Every practitioner should have several such favorable commentaries. Chances are we could also obtain testimonials from patients of orthopedic surgeons who helped where chiropractic failed. The controversy between established medicine and chiropractic is not the subject of this book. The point made in Peggy's case, and in mine, is that the muscle testing of applied kinesiology helped isolate a basic cause so it could be properly treated.

I have experienced the handicraft of seven different chiropractors, from at least three chiropractic schools or philosophies, two osteopaths, a naprapath, and a muscular friend who 'knew how' to fix an upper back that 'went out.'

I have had my breath literally knocked out of me as the physician crunched down on the vertebrae in the middle of my back with all the force he could muster. I have worn large lifts in my shoes — one had me lift the left heel, another the right heel a few years later.

I was told by my late father (who drank coffee, as I did) that my lower back pain was a congenital lumbar condition I inherited from him. He had the same lower back pain for more years than I, and I'd bet a serious wager his right sartorius would test weak, just like mine. Like father like son!

I was shown X-ray pictures of my spine showing a curved and crooked column of vertebrae.

Regardless of the skill of the practitioner I consulted whenever my back or neck would 'go out,' leaving me in great pain and practically immobile, the results were the same. I would be pushed, pulled, clackety-clicked, and charged. The intense pain would subside, slowly, and I would return to my normal chronic lower-back-pain state, which I'd learned to tune out most of the time. It woke me every morning without fail, however, and would not 'tune out' until I got out of bed and moved around.

Using muscle testing and AK's 'vertebral challenge' procedures, Dr Hetrick needed about five sessions to return my overweight, forty-eight-year-old structure to a balanced state. In the process I experienced some pretty painful sensations in certain muscles, but when the smoke cleared, the culprit was gone. The pains were not from the manipulations *per se* — manipulations are generally painless — but from old muscles learning some new, more balanced tricks.

While it has been generally accepted for a long time that subluxations can cause various and sundry health problems throughout the body, the knowledge of exactly how they do it is theoretical.

Dr Walther's text tells how one system of spinal adjustment developed from a diagnosis of the health problem and a study of nerve distribution. The early researchers manipulated particular vertebrae they assumed were associated with the condition and hoped it would solve the problem. Walther calls this a 'cookbook approach.'

Later schools of structural manipulation strove to locate areas along the spinal column that appeared to be malfunctioning in order to determine the location of the subluxation. Then these experimenters adjusted the spine, regardless of the patient's other symptoms. This practice eventually proved to be an advancement because the correlation between a specific symptom and spinal subluxations does not always match perfectly. For example, a stomach disorder does not have to be related to a subluxation, even though both conditions may exist in a patient.

Dr Walther also discusses X-ray evaluation of the spine:

The direction for corrective adjustment of the vertebra is often determined by x-ray evaluation of the spine. Although this has been a valuable method of determining corrective procedures, it leaves much to be desired because: 1) if actual spinal column changes are made, the x-ray quickly becomes obsolete for the patient's current condition; 2) re-evaluation by x-ray gives the patient unwanted radiation; 3) congenital anomalies [little irregularities you are born with] such as the assymetric development of articular processes [parts of vertebrae], can lead the valuation astray; and 4) most x-ray evaluation used today is static evaluation, which does not take into account the dynamic function of the body.

Despite the drawbacks, X-ray is necessary on a limited basis to help the physician observe for trauma, congenital anomalies, and pathology such as osteoporosis, arthritis, infections, and malignancy.

All chiropractors are well schooled in the procedure called palpation. Palpation means examining by touch, in this case feeling the groups of muscles along the spine in order to evaluate the spinal condition. The sense of touch is highly trained in all AK physicians.

When Dr Hetrick palpated and adjusted my spine he manually tested a leg muscle while I lay face down. He would finger the muscles around a particular vertebra, then either push or pull a little of this and a little of that. Then he would quickly test the leg muscle for strength or weakness, to learn whether his adjustments had been appropriate. He was employing the vertebral challenge developed by Dr Goodheart in 1972. This technique has the following advantages, according to Dr Walther's text:

1.   It determines exactly which vertebra is subluxated.

2.   The precise direction of correction is revealed, regardless of whether the correction is on one plane only, or a combination of three planes.

3.   After a corrective attempt is made, the vertebra can be re-tested immediately to determine whether the attempt resulted in an effective correction.

4.   The patient may easily be tested in several positions and after specific types of activity, such as walking or running, or other dynamic motions, thus testing him the way he lives rather than lying on an x-ray table or an adjusting table for the physician's convenience.

5.   The patient can be re-evaluated each time he returns to the office, thus giving dynamic information as his structural balance changes and the spinal mechanism makes adaptations to the change.

As mentioned earlier, the triad-of-health concept lends itself to the now-proved notion that one aspect of health may affect the others. A chemical imbalance can cause a muscle weakness that leads to a subluxation. A trauma can cause a subluxation that chemically leads to a glandular misfunction. Emotional stress can set the process in motion as well.

The body is a self-correcting, self-healing mechanism. Dr Walther points out that it 'stands to reason that many more subluxations are corrected by the body itself than by doctors in any field.'

The spinal column is supported by various muscles as shown in Figures 9-13. These diagrams will give you an idea of muscle placement and of the balances required to keep your spine in optimum position.

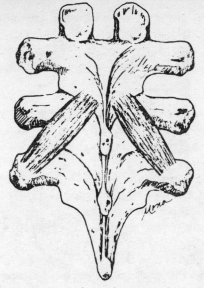

Figure 9.   Balanced rotatores longus.

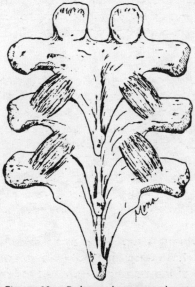

Figure 10.   Balanced rotatores brevis.

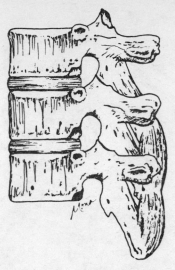

Figure 11. Balanced interspinalis muscles.

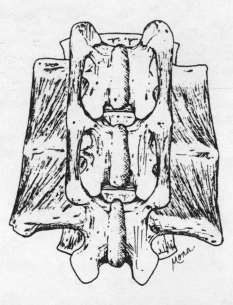

Figure 12. Balanced intertransversarii muscles.

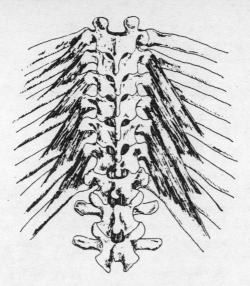

Figure 13. Balanced levatores costarum muscles.

Applied kinesiology has added an important dimension to the art of spinal manipulation, and we predict that within the next decade it will become a standard method of diagnosis and evaluation for all structural therapy. With continued research, it is likely that the nutritional/chemical aspects of manual muscle testing will also be accepted generally.

Chapter Seven:

Proprioceptors — Muscle Communicators

The complaint of nagging backache associated with standing up for prolonged periods of time is at one time or another voiced in practically every household. Although it is a common complaint, the probable cause of the ache is not generally known. Chances are that the AK practitioner is more conversant with this painful muscle-nerve phenomenon than any other physician. The distress in the extensor muscles in the back of the spine, expressed as nagging pain felt by persons who remain on their feet for a long time — even in well-fitting shoes — is more often than not caused by faulty signals sent out to the rest of the body by the muscles of the feet. This is because the proprioceptors (tiny nerve centers) in the muscles of the feet and ankles can garble their signals to the rest of the body.

We are dealing with tiny but sensitive groups of nerve cells capable of complex communication regarding bodily encounters with the myriad stimuli in the environment. Applied kinesiology has shown that faulty nerve communication from proprioceptors, especially those in the muscles of the feet, can cause problems elsewhere in the body. Neurophysiologists have done the most research to isolate, understand, and classify the component parts of the proprioceptive system. However, AK physicians have assumed the leadership role in clinical application and practical knowledge of proprioceptors and what they mean to better health and physical condition.

Before delving into the application of diagnosis and therapies involving proprioceptors, we'll try to make it clear just what proprioceptors are, and what they do. The reason this is a formidable task is that the complexity and interaction of reflex activity defies total understanding within current levels of electrophysiology ability,' according to Dr Walther. We already touched on the complexity of electrophysiology when we explained 'energy patterns.' How molecules and cells use the multifaceted phenomena of the electromagnetic spectrum is only partially understood, but more is being discovered on a daily basis by researchers around the world.

To get an idea of the complexity, one research paper states: 'On each spinal cord motoneuron [tiny nerve cell] there are approximately 6,000 synaptic terminations [like female electric outlets in the wall capable of accepting plugs]. In considering reflex activity, even a seemingly simple event such as the monosynaptic response [single synapse or connection between a cell and nerve impulse], which results from projection of a sensory fiber onto a motoneuron, must be viewed as a product of the whole nervous system and not just one isolated input-output pathway.'

Because applied kinesiology evaluates all of the interactions within the body, Dr Walther states, 'The effort is directed toward finding the signaling mechanism which is causing the dysfunction and eliminating its source to return the body to predictable organization. Thus, the effort directed to the proprioceptors is to locate and eliminate stimulation which causes volleys of impulses that are misdirected.'

Many conditions in our bodies are now recognized as due to improper signaling from proprioceptors located in the muscles, tendons, joints, skin and fascia (tissues), or those proprioceptors designed for orientation in space (inner ear). Seasickness would be a common example of such a condition; lower back pain from a rotated pelvis caused by improper messages signaled by muscles in the feet is another.

Researchers have isolated three kinds of proprioceptors — the muscle proprioceptors, proprioceptors of the joints and skin, and the equilibirium proprioceptors. Each of these groups has within its components equipment capable of 'phasic or tonic' activity. Phasic refers to stimuli that travels through stages, like from hot to cold, and tonic refers to tone quality such as hardness and softness.

One gets a semblance of the idea of proprioceptive

communication when considering the numerous aspects of the sense of touch. Nerve sensors can tell us hot, cold, warm, moist, dry, hard, soft, slimy, thick, thin, coarse, smooth, etc. even though we may be blindfolded. Of course, such sensory ability is not limited to just our fingers, but we can sense by touching with any part of our bodies.

When a competent AK physician pushes gently on portions of a muscle, or pulls segments of muscle apart during his session on your body, he knows how and where to activate nerve receptors in order to gauge the nature of particular complaints. Muscle nerve receptors are equipped with tiny neuromuscular spindles and the Golgi tendon organ. The spindles influence the activity of the muscle in which they reside; they also influence, with outgoing signals, various synergistic and antagonistic muscles elsewhere in the body — muscles that work with and against the spindle's muscle. The Golgi tendon organ is designed to inhibit the muscle housing the tendon, its nerve receptors working to produce the opposite effect on a muscle from that produced by the spindle.

These electrophysiological receptors in your joints and skin vary in their types and are designed to automatically signal muscles into position when you move around. The skin receptors, in addition to responding to the many variations of the sense of touch, are also influential in muscle reflex actions (knee jerk, for example) and at the same time help give you a clear sense of your position in space — standing, lying down, rolling, standing on your head and so forth. Gymnasts, acrobats and divers have highly trained or conditioned position receptors. We take this marvellous system for granted, of course, but contemplating how the body communicates and copes with the myriad sensory stimuli of our environment, and does so constantly, should make us respect nature's handiwork all the more.

The ear and neck area proprioceptors are of tremendous importance in the structural balance of the body and for our orientation in space. By understanding the mechanism of these receptors and their influence on posture, the AK physician has greater insight into many problems of vertebral fixations and upper cervical orientation with the skull, plus clues to cranial/sacral dysfunction — all of which may be responsible for structural imbalances.

Perhaps it is time the scions of medical science give chiropractic and applied kinesiology their due. For example, when the U.S. space program ran into considerable difficulty attempting to prepare men for the weightless environment of outer space, the established medical professionals were unsure that certain orientation problems would be overcome, but a chiropractor, knowledgeable about proprioceptors, helped design the space suits so the astronauts' bodies could easily cope with the stresses of blasting off into weightlessness.

When Dr Hetrick first manipulated my lower spine and straightened my pelvis, among other things, he stretched and squeezed the proprioceptors in my spinal muscles to help him further determine the essential cause of my years of lower back pain. The pressure of his fingertips was causing my neuromuscular spindle cells to influence certain reactive muscles and weaken them. The object was to loosen tight muscles that were pulling my spine out of position. What often happens to people when a muscle proprioceptor gets its signal crossed and garbles communication is that a reactive muscle influenced by that particular transmitter either weakens or tightens, having a sort of domino effect on the structure.

Spindle cells in the muscles are heavily concentrated in the abdomen muscles, but are found in every muscle in the body. The functioning of these bioelectrical receptors/transmitters is entirely unconscious — we don't feel a thing, unless the signals get crossed up and cause problems. These spindles are relatively easy for the AK physician to manipulate and test, or therapy-localize. However, the other muscle receptors, the Golgi tendon organs, are much more mysterious and difficult for the physicians to locate and properly palpate or manipulate.

Evidently the Golgi tendon organs were hard to find in the first place. You will get a good idea of how your AK physician examines Golgi tendon organs from reading this section taken directly from Dr Walther's textbook:

As on the neuromuscular spindle cell, the influence of manual manipulation of the Golgi tendon can be observed by influencing normally functioning Golgi tendon organs. The only difficulty in performing this experiment is in applying the manipulative force at the correct location. It requires excellent palpatory skills to find where the Golgi tendon organ is probably located, and a certain amount of luck that the receptor is actually there. This is necessary because a normal Golgi tendon organ will not therapy localize, revealing its location. To cause a strong muscle to weaken in a normal subject, digital pressure is applied over the probable location of the Golgi tendon organ in alignment with the muscle fibers away from the belly of the muscle. If the attempt is successful, there will be an immediate dramatic weakening of the muscle which will last from approximately a half-minute to several minutes. In attempting this experiment, a muscle should be selected which does not have an extensive amount of tendon surface area, and the muscle should have adequate strength so that it is not easily overpowered. A good muscle to use is the rectur femoris of the quadriceps group [the long muscle making up the front of your thigh, running from hip to knee]. The entire quadriceps group is more difficult for achieving successful weakening because of the larger area of origin of the muscles.

The neuromuscular spindles monitor the length of the muscle, while the Golgi tendon organs monitor the tensions of the muscles. The inhibitory nature of the Golgi tendon organ's communications is a built-in safety factor for our bodies. Sometimes signals get crossed or we exert too much conscious pressure, and damage is done, such as muscle tears or pulls, tendon damage and ligament tears. Athletes are familiar with many such structural problems. Again, Dr Walther's text provides some interesting insight:

Many muscles have much greater strength potential than the structure can withstand. A failure of muscle control can cause possible avulsion or tearing of the muscle itself. Stimulation to the Golgi tendon organ inhibits the muscle from going past its structural capabilities. An example of the effectiveness of the Golgi tendon apparatus may be found in observing individuals arm wrestling. The loser generally gives out completely — all at once — when impulses from the Golgi tendon organ overpower the alpha motor neuron impulses and shut the muscle down. It is observed, however, that many trained weightlifters apparently have learnt to mentally override the Golgi tendon mechanism to provide a greater amount of strength potential. This can, of course, be structurally damaging to the body, as in the situation when an arm wrestler fractures the humerus.

It seems to us that no other medical speciality has the expertise to deal with athletic stresses, strains and injuries more properly than applied kinesiology. While AK practitioners cannot do the surgery, they can certainly thoroughly ascertain whether surgery is necessary in many cases, and manual muscle testing is certainly helpful in aiding an athlete who is recovering from an injury. To my way of thinking, it would pay the orthopedic surgeons and athletic trainers to learn the art of applied kinesiology. At least it would certainly pay the patients for these specialists to do so.

To put all the technical data about proprioceptors into perspective, Dr Hetrick provided an on-table demonstration of how one muscle's nerve centers will affect the strength or weakness, tension or relaxation of another associated with it. I had been undergoing the therapy-localization processes for my coffee-weakened adrenals and my right sartorius was tense from the strain. The sartorius is the long upper leg muscle running from pelvis to knee down the inside of the thigh, which is used when muscle-testing the adrenal glands' function.

'To weaken or relax a muscle,' Dr Hetrick explained, 'the proprioceptors are pressed together, like this.' With that, he pressured the center of my sartorius with his thumb and fingers and the tension vanished from the muscle.

'Now, the quadraceps is reactive to the sartorius, and all the nervous energy utilized by your tense sartorius has undoubtedly weakened your quadraceps.'

He tested the quadraceps, which runs down the front of the thigh from pelvis to knee, and it was, indeed, weak. Then he pulled the center portion of the long muscle apart with his fingers. To weaken a muscle the proprioceptors are pressured inward between the fingers, to strengthen, they are stretched apart by the fingers (see Figures 14-17). Sure enough, after he finished, the quadraceps tested strong.

An applied kinesiologist can weaken any muscle he chooses, and he can manipulate the various muscles that are reactive or associated with particular muscles in order to demonstrate the communications between muscle proprioceptors. Dr Hetrick abandoned my right leg and took up my left leg, which was as normal as one could expect, and deliberately pressured the quadraceps proprioceptors causing that powerful leg muscle to weaken considerably. Of course, it had already been demonstrated to me that by merely massaging certain lymphatic reflex points, or by touching specific acupuncture points, the muscles affected by those points would strengthen or weaken. Dr Hetrick flashed me a satisfied grin and reiterated: 'The body is a completely integrated complex of systems — circulatory, lymph, nervous, structural and acupuncture meridians. One cannot stimulate one system without affecting each of the others in some way. Understanding this and using the knowledge to help patients is the goal of the holistic physician.'

In the beginning of this chapter on muscle proprioceptors, which are the key to AK muscle-testing procedures, we called attention to the many complaints people have when they have been on their feet for prolonged periods. It is the integration of the body systems that leads to many of the pains and miseries people suffer needlessly because they are not acquainted with the theories and practice of applied kinesiology. A waitress, whose job keeps her on her feet for long hours at a time, may complain of headache and stiffness in her neck and shoulders at the end of the day, even though her feet are not particularly pained. The odds are the headache and neck pains stem from her feet because of the nature of muscle proprioceptors.

Dr Walther's brochures cover this problem area thoroughly and

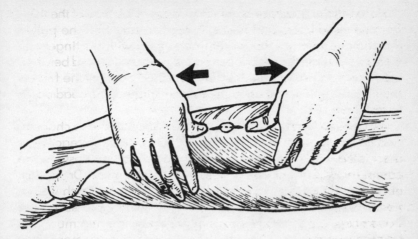

Figure 14. Direction of digital pressure to strengthen muscle which is weak from apparent neuro-muscular spindle malfunction.

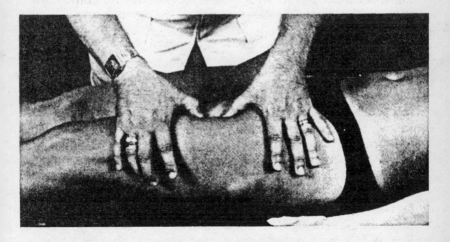

Figure 15. Representative location of neuromuscular spindle and pressure application for strengthening rectus femoris muscle.

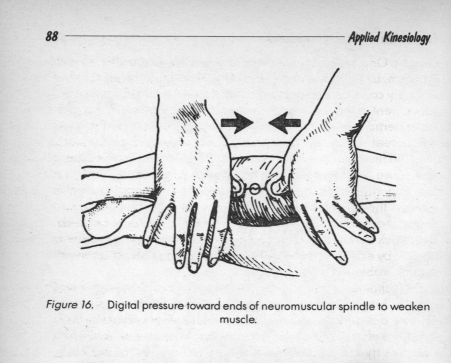

Figure 16. Digital pressure toward ends of neuromuscular spindle to weaken muscle.

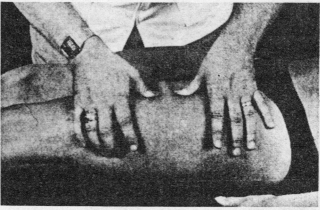

Figure 17. Representative location for digital pressure on ends of neuromuscular spindle to weaken muscle. Press together.

clearly. One of his brochures is entitled 'Whatever the Health Problem, Look to Your Feet — They May Have the Answer.' Another is simply called 'Foot Pronation.' Pronation is the term for an inward movement of the ankle and the flattening of the arch in the foot. It's extremely common, even in this age of runners and joggers whose feet and ankles might be expected to be strong and straight.

In the first of the two brochures, Dr Walther writes, 'Foot problems can cause health problems in any part of your body — and your feet may not even hurt.' He then adds that many people will also express the complaint that 'When my feet hurt, I hurt all over!' Our feet and ankles, it seems, are good for chiropractic business. Dr Hetrick admits that foot problems ranked alongside problems caused by eating too much refined sugar among his patients with 'spine' problems.

Dr Walther points out that recent research in chiropractic and applied kinesiology has discovered that the proprioceptors in the feet are designed to communicate to every other part of the body the sense of body movement and position. When we walk all kinds of nerve messages are being signaled to the rest of the body, especially to the shoulders (see Figure 18). 'This information causes the muscles in the back of the shoulder to relax, allowing the arm to move smoothly forward in synchronization,' Walther writes.

The research into the 'gait mechanism,' or 'walking gait,' would amaze you with the amount of detailed study that's gone into the simple procedure of walking. In order to find out how something can go wrong because something is amiss in one's walking gait, the researchers had to first determine what a 'normal walk' consists of. Experiments on gait, using equipment other than just observation, were first conducted in Germany in 1836. During the intervening century and a half the research equipment has become sophisticated and computerized. Gait studies today use a 'Grafpen sonic digitizer' to obtain a computer readout, a plot, electromyograms (readings similar to lie detector readings) and motion pictures to analyze throughout a walking cycle the precise rotations of the lower extremity joints from every angle, the length of step, the cadence, the walking velocity and the duration of weight on one foot relative to the complete cycle. Researchers,

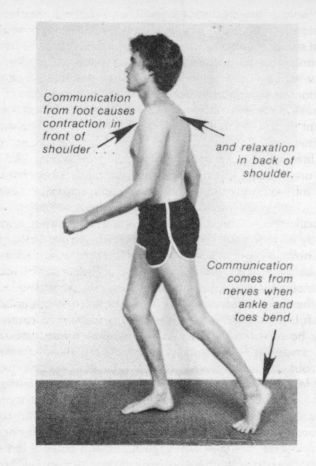

Figure 18. Demonstration of how nerve messages from the foot have far-ranging effects.

and not only AK practitioners, have learned a great deal from these studies. Psychiatrists, for example, have found that normal persons propel themselves forward when they walk while depressed patients walk with a lifting motion of the leg without much forward momentum.

'The scientific concepts of gait have added totally new dimensions to our examination of patients,' Dr Hetrick said. 'At a recent seminar with Dr Goodheart, we learned that 45 percent of humanity takes a longer step with the left foot; 45 percent step longer with the right foot and only 10 percent of the people take equidistant or so-called normal steps.'

Because people walk every day, the effects of walking are pertinent to everyone's health. Dr Walther's brochure points out that if the foot is not functioning normally, from a previous injury, or flat feet, or hammertoes, or dropped metatarsals, etc., 'the nerves are stimulated in a confused manner and do not send correct information to the shoulder for harmonious muscular action.'

Try walking and swinging your arms the opposite of normal. The body is working against itself, isn't it? Trying to walk out of synchronization for any length of time is difficult to do and cumbersome, but one doesn't have to exaggerate the motions to experience problems such as aching joints or muscle fatigue. Just having the shoulder and arm moving slightly out of synchronization is stressful. The problem does not stop with simple strain and fatigue, however. With every step, every movement, there are countless nerve impulses exchanging electrochemical information throughout your entire body. When the messages from the foot and ankle are confused or garbled a result can be pain. Dr Walther puts it this way: 'Many symptoms can result. As the neck becomes strained and fatigued from poor body economy, the small nerves going through the muscular areas of the base of the skull become irritated; headaches may develop around the base of the skull and radiate over the head. Upper back strain may eventually cause a vertebral misalignment which irritates the nerves exiting between the vertebrae. This may possibly cause digestive disturbances or other health problems from the subsequent autonomic nervous system imbalance.'

With all of our weight coming down on our feet with every step we take, it is no wonder the problems that can be derived keep chiropractors in business. 'People tend to neglect their feet,' according to Dr Hetrick, 'and the feet probably take more abuse than any other part of the body.'

One of the first things Dr Hetrick did for me was wrap my feet and ankles as though I were an athlete preparing for a contest. The wrappings were to be left on for three or four days in order to help my foot muscles get back to normal and to stop sending garbled nerve messages to my upper back and neck. While my lower back pains were found to be related to diet (caffeine) and the weakening of my body energy systems related to the weary adrenal glands, the pains in my upper back and neck related directly to my feet. For years, prior to discovering applied kinesiology, I had periodically felt the vertebrae in my upper back, well up between my shoulder blades, 'go out,' and when a certain one finally clicked, causing a sharp pain and preventing me from moving my head and neck freely, I would seek a chiropractor for an 'adjustment.' In recent years, perhaps the last five, the period between sharp pains had diminished from six months to six weeks. It not only hurt, and made me ineffective, but it was costly to return to a physician every six weeks or so.

Dr Hetrick not only wrapped my feet, but he fitted me for 'orthodics,' which are supports designed to be placed in the shoes under the feet. First, I had to make a mold of my feet with my weight evenly distributed in a casting of soft polystyrene foam. The molds were sent to experts who used them to fashion the supports on which I now stand. The improvement was immediately noticeable. Previously my back would give out if I had to walk more than a few blocks on cement. Dress shoes hurt my feet if I had to walk in them more than a few hundred yards. Running shoes and tennis shoes caused me less pain than dress shoes, but one healthy set of tennis left my legs and back cramped for up to twenty-four hours. Following the insertion of the molded supports, which helped my feet muscle proprioceptors keep their messages straight, every phase of walking and running exhibited considerable improvement.

The orthodics are not necessarily 'lifts' designed to correct leg length irregularities, but they can be.

Dr Walther's brochures feature clear illustrations of the warning signs of foot problems. (see Figure 19). He lists the indications of foot problems as: 'Imbalanced shoe wear, corns, shoe breakbrown, burning feet, calluses, numbness, leg pain, hammertoe position, leg fatigue, poor circulation, bunions and foot pronation.'

The foot pronation brochure is brief and to the point:

The foot is a marvel of structural design. When functioning normally, it endures a tremendous amount of shock throughout the day and still smiles at day's end, with no evidence of fatigue. Unfortunately, this is not true for a large number of people. Foot problems are very common. Interestingly, when the foot is involved, the entire body usually becomes involved as a result.

The most common foot problem is that of pronation. Foot pronation means that some of the bones of the foot have rolled inward, causing the foot to lose its structural integrity and placing strain in the foot and ankle as they function.

Foot pronation can often be seen as the inward movement of the ankle, and also as the flattening of the arch. The arch does not always flatten; however, there will always be strain beneath it as the individual stands.

It is relatively easy to observe foot pronation [see Figure 20].

Foot pronation is aggravated as a result of poor strength in the muscles supporting the ankle and the bottom of the foot. This is not usually due to lack of physical exercise of the muscles; rather, it is interference with the muscle's controlling mechanisms. For example, there may be interference with the nerve which causes contraction. The illustrations [see Figure 21] show some of the muscles involved in foot and ankle stability. You will note that a number of the muscles are in the calf of the leg.

The primary causes of foot pronation are (a) an inadequately treated ankle strain — in other words, it was only treated with rest and no attention was paid to the muscular support; (b) improper shoes, and (c) injury to the foot.

Dr Walther concludes the brochure with statements about having the doctor of chiropractic who is knowledgeable in applied kinesiology test the muscles and perhaps prescribe specific exercises for the muscles in the sole of the foot. He describes

Figure 19.   The warning signs of foot problems.

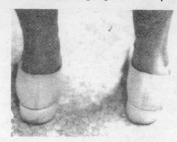

SHOE WEAR

Heels should wear to the back and slightly to the side. Sole wear should be even. The back (counter) of the shoe should not break down or roll over.

DEVELOPING HAMMERTOES

Hammertoes develop as a result of muscular imbalance in the foot and leg. If treated early enough, they can be corrected.

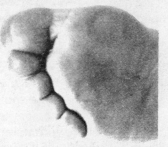

CALLUS FORMATION

There should be no calluses on the bottom or top of the foot. Callus formation on the bottom is due to poor weight bearing by the foot. On top, the formation is usually due to poor shoe fit; it can be from poor foot position.

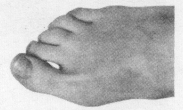

BUNIONS

Bunions may develop from improper shoe fit, and especially from foot breakdown and muscular imbalance. Early treatment produces good results unless there is a congenital muscle deformity.

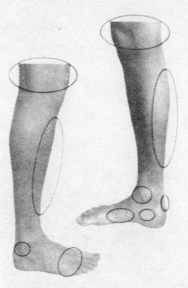

PAIN LOCATIONS

There should be no pain in the foot, ankle, or leg upon pressure. Press or poke into your hand and compare the sensation with that of pressing or poking into your foot. If the foot is much more tender, it's likely that there is a problem in the foot-ankle complex, affecting your health.

Figure 20. means of testing for pronation of the foot.

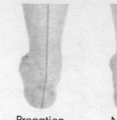

Pronation   Normal

When standing, there should be an alignment of the Achilles tendon with the calf of the leg.

When standing, no weight should be placed into the medial longitudinal arch of the foot.

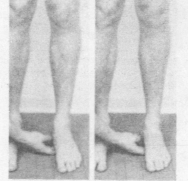

Relaxed stance   Rotated leg

There should be minimal tension in the 'arch' area of the foot when standing. Have someone check for this by placing his finger beneath your foot in the arch area and feeling the tension. Then rotate your knee outward, keeping your foot in place; check to see if the tension is relaxed. If there is a significant lessening of tension under your foot, pronation is present.

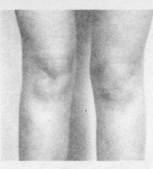

Internal rotation of the knees is an indication of foot pronation. When standing in a relaxed manner, check the position of the kneecap; it should be in the center of the knee. If the knee is in internal rotation, the kneecap will be toward the midline.

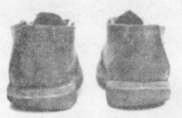

Check a pair of shoes you've worn for some time. The heel should wear toward the back and slightly to the side. The counter, or back portion of the shoe, should stay aligned with the heel. Your shoes should wear in a balanced manner, and not 'run over.'

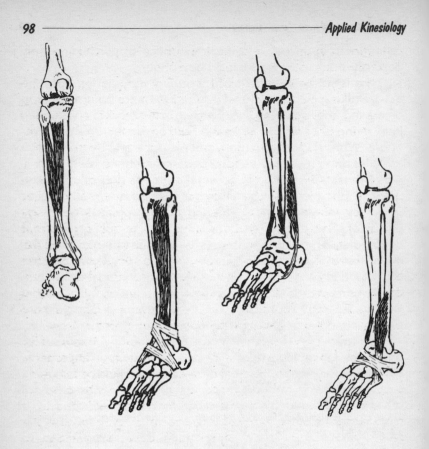

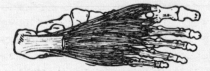

Figure 21. Some of the muscles involved in foot and ankle stability.

orthodics or supports, and the importance of purchasing only perfectly fitting and well constructed shoes.

There is yet another problem area that may derive from the act of walking. Perhaps you have heard warnings against running or jogging, especially jogging, because of the shock to one's system just having one's weight strike the hard pavement over and over again. While it's true that many people appear to be able to run for miles over pavement without seeming to suffer adverse effects, the truth is that any tiny abnormality in one's gait or stride can produce 'dural torque.' The subject of dural torque really excites Dr Hetrick, who has a special feeling for how applied kinesiology can be of service to athletes. The term 'dural torque' comes from dura mater, a hard, tough, fibrous membrane that makes up the outermost of three coverings protecting the spinal cord and the brain, and from the word describing the mechanical action that produces rotation. Whenever you tighten a nut on a bolt with a wrench, you are torquing the nut. The dura mater is durable, hard material and it is stiff enough to accept forces of torque. However, while torque is fine for nuts and bolts, it is painfully improper for our spines, let alone our brains. If you jog, walk or run improperly, which can occur for any number of reasons, you could be torqueing your dura mater and paying a price. Many times a spinal subluxation caused by this torquing has been adjusted by a chiropractor or other manipulative specialist, only to have the professional manipulation ruined by the patient's continuing to walk, run or jog improperly and continuing to torque the dura mater.

The key is to be carefully examined by a competent AK physician to make sure there are no previously undisclosed wrinkles in your gait mechanism. In my case, Dr Hetrick not only wrapped my feet and ankles on several occasions, and provided me with custom-molded foot supports, he also strove to have me improve my previous torqueing condition by having me take a longer stride with my right leg when I walked. A little concentration on daily exercise walks makes it easy to overcome the silly feeling of striding unnaturally. After several weeks of this walking therapy, my lower back pains had vanished altogether and there was far less need to visit the chiropractor.

How Dr Hetrick knew to have me stride out with the right leg instead of the left was a matter of clinical experience and detailed training in AK procedures. In about 70 percent of American patients the right leg is slightly longer than the left. Curiously, Japanese researchers have found exactly the opposite — 70 percent of the Japanese have slightly longer left legs. There is also considerable evidence that the Japanese use their right brain more than Americans or Europeans. There appears to be a correlation between the phenomenon of left brain/right brain, which is discussed in the next chapter on body organization, and the slightly longer leg phenomenon. In my case, I fell within the majority of the statistical range, and my right leg was indeed slightly longer. Dr Hetrick determined this fact by turning my feet inward with his hand, one after the other, and observing my body reactions. In addition to the foot twisting procedure, he muscle-tested his way up and down my spine double-checking my pelvis and sacroiliac for signs of dural torsion.

'Dural torque may not result in a major skeletal distortion,' Hetrick explained, 'but it's nothing to ignore or remain ignorant of. As Dr Goodheart explained, the dura mater is exceptionally hard — you can hang a person's body on the stuff and it won't stretch. When it starts to torque or rotate it can compress in one spinal area and cause tension in another at the same time. This can disturb the function of the spinal fluid.'

Since my right foot turned in more readily than my left during the test procedure, that was the leg designated for the longer strides. The exercise was designed to counter previous dural torque. The competent AK physician will have several special muscle-testing procedures to determine the extent of dural torque and which exercises are suited to the patient's particular problem.

Problems in the spine caused by dural torque could have been caused by improper nerve signals from proprioceptors in the feet. We have already seen that there may be many variations in the condition of the feet and the gait mechanism, but that's not the whole of it when it comes to proprioceptors. Research has indicated that nutrition may also be a factor in correcting improper signaling by muscle proprioceptors. Dr Goodheart's research led him to believe the enzyme phosphatase, which is found in raw bone concentrate and raw potato and protein concentrate, is a key nutrition for helping the body overcome dysfunctioning muscle proprioceptors. Muscle-testing procedures indicate that raw bone concentrate, indeed, helps correct proprioceptive problems that persist.

More is known about the muscle proprioceptors than about the skin and joint proprioceptors, but ongoing research indicates there is a far more important role for the skin proprioceptors than previously anticipated by medical science. This new learning may bode well for the advocates of the 'touch' therapies now gaining in popularity in the U.S. Apparently, there is a growing body of clinical evidence that the skin receptors and the joint receptors have a widespread general effect on the entire muscular system. Dr Goodheart says that more research is needed on reaction to skin receptor stimuli. I wonder if additional research might unveil a strong correlation between skin proprioceptors and the seemingly mysterious abilities of acupuncture to demonstrate heretofore unexplained physical phenomena — such as its ability to provide a form of general anesthesia.

Noted anthropologist Ashley Montagu has commented on the intricacy and potency of skin receptors. He wrote that 'the skin itself does not think, but its sensitivity is so great . . . that for versatility it must be ranked second only to the brain itself.' Montagu pointed out that the skin has the ability to pick up and transmit an extraordinarily wide variety of signals and make a wide range of responses, exceeding all other sense organs in that respect. Drs Walther, Goodheart and Hetrick all feel that the skin has not received the attention it deserves from physiologists. Applied kinesiology is the only discipline currently incorporating the functions of skin receptors in all diagnostic evaluations, even though the medical literature devotes but meager attention to the exact mechanisms of skin proprioceptors and their role in body integration.

Early in the book we stressed that it would be a good practice for parents of young babies to bring their offspring to an AK physician for examination. Few things may be more important to a rapidly developing child than the proper conditioning of proprioceptive responses.

Chapter Eight:

Body Organization:
Right Brain/Left Brain

A fascinating area of research during the past twenty years has been the study of the influence of left-brain/right-brain dominance within individuals. We average folk read much about this brain-hemisphere dominance telling whether we are flighty or practical, whether we prefer accounting or painting. Well, that's scratching the surface of this particular aspect of body organization, which is the third major arena for AK manual muscle-testing, following structural organization and chemical-nutritional organization.

Our nervous system controls our body organization without any help from our conscious mind. The endocrine system, which secretes hormones (chemical messengers) into the bloodstream upon command from specific nerves, is a secondary control system to the central nervous system. If for some reason the signals get messed up, like faulty proprioceptor signals, the body reaction may be messed up and too much or too little hormone is released. Sometimes the signals simply aren't sent, or they are sent to a wrong address in the body, or the addressee can't understand the message. Whatever the reasons, when the body's organizational system of nerves and hormones is disturbed, the result is disorganization.

Applied kinesiologists call such disorganization 'switching,' and refer to patients exhibiting symptoms of confused body organization as being 'switched.' For example, Carole's son Sam is an excellent tennis player who has shown natural co-ordination for the game without ever having lessons. However, there are times when his co-ordination abandons him and he can barely co-ordinate well enough to serve the ball slowly into the correct quadrant of the court. It's as though his right and left sides have quit communicating and co-ordinating — and that's exactly what occurs in his body organization. In Sam's case evaluations by an applied kinesiologist showed him that the chemicals in beer triggered his body disorganization. He also learned that certain rock music sounds also triggered his switching condition, which confused his left-brain/right-brain organization. Since discovering these trigger mechanisms, Sam has avoided them and has not suffered recurrences. Most of us sustain some symptoms of switching, but few experience switching as severely as Sam's case.

The phenomenon of body organization begins quite early, according to researchers; however, the experts are not so clear on what begins when. Fetuses have been shown to suck their fingers, respond to noise, etc. Certain muscle abilities are innate. Nevertheless, the moment we are brought into the world we begin conditioning, training, educating and co-ordinating our body organization. Infants wiggle their fingers, wave their arms, suckle at their mothers' breasts, crane their necks, and so forth. Every movement is repeated thousands of times, thereby educating the nerves and muscles. Crawling, walking and running are all part and parcel of acquired body organization. AK physicians believe that babies should definitely crawl before they learn to walk, that if a baby somehow scoots both legs together without co-ordinating the left-right movement of crawling, or if the infant is placed in a 'walker' before having the opportunity to learn to crawl, it's quite likely the individual will grow up with body disorganization problems.

Our bodies have two halves operating the brain and nerve control centers. The right side of the brain controls the left side of the body and the left side of the brain operates the right side of the body — an X pattern intended by nature. After five to eight years of childhood activity the crossing mechanisms are generally established and traits of dominance are developed. Left-handedness or right-handedness are the most commonly recognized evidences of the dominance of one hemisphere in an individual's body organization. Pediatricians today know much more about the nature of body organizational development and efforts are made to educate parents to the pitfalls of any interference with natural development. Years ago it was quite common for parents to attempt to educate a child away from a tendency toward left-handedness. Such manipulation can cause body disorganization, perhaps to an extent leading to severe health problems. Improper crossing and anything inhibiting naturally developed dominance, whether through intentional manipulation, or caused by childhood injury or a major trauma at any time in life, can cause a full spectrum of symptoms. Children may have difficulty learning, be clumsy or hyperactive due to body disorganization. Adults may develop muscle spasms, spinal subluxations and an inability to hold chiropractic adjustments, among other general conditions.

Dr Hetrick says that a large portion of the applied kinesiology practice is devoted to evaluating for abnormal body organization. He explains, 'Body disorganization can be caused by many things including poor nutrition, allergic reaction, environmental pollution, stress or trauma. The symptoms may be simple, like a spinal discomfort or excessive fatigue at the end of a day, or it may be serious resulting in pathology such as deteriorating an organ or gland.'

Unchecked body disorganization caused by faulty signals arising from a seemingly minor injury may cause problems years later. We have Dr Hetrick's example, given earlier, of a patient whose ankle injury resulted in a foot subluxation, which caused improper signals to be sent by her foot proprioceptors. The faulty nerve signals resulted in chronic headache and back pain in her case. In other instances Dr Hetrick has noted cases where faulty nerve signals resulted in poor co-ordination of the gait mechanism and inhibited the neck and shoulder muscles. At first the patients experienced mere tension in the shoulders and discomfort, but as the condition persisted the result was inflammation or bursitis. In some cases, when the condition continues long enough, there will be likely involvement of the knee and hip joints, possibly leading to arthritic conditions.

The strength of applied kinesiology lies in the ability to muscle-test and therapy-localize until the basic causes of a particular symptom are ferreted out. The processes involved in discovering hidden contributors to pain or pathology utilize a growing body of knowledge of body language as it relates to muscle-testing and the triad of health-structure, chemistry and mentality.

To determine whether the disorganization is structural, the AK physician is taught to interpret reflexes or signals sent from your inner ear, your vision and the complex muscle and joint proprioceptors located where the head meets the neck. The sternocleidomastoid muscle (see Figure 22) and upper trapezius

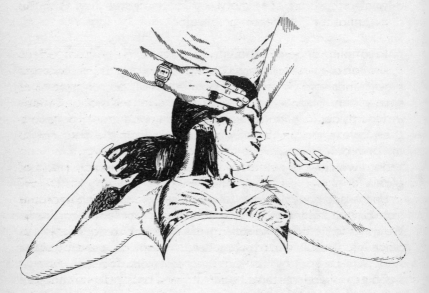

Figure 22. The sternocleidomastoid and upper trapezius muscles.

muscles, when tested, will reveal to the applied kinesiologist nerve organization information from both the spinal cord and the brain. When I was being muscle-tested and evaluated, Dr Hetrick instructed me to turn my head to the left and aim my eyes to the right. Then he requested the reverse — head right, eyes left. Had the muscle he was testing suddenly weakened, it would have indicated body disorganization from a structural cause.

Dr Walther explains that inner ear and visual righting reflexes are cranial in nature and that if a 'cranial fault or cervical subluxation exists, and there is conflict between the cranial nerve and the spinal nerve supply to these muscles,' referring to the muscles around the joints of the upper neck. His textbook reads:

Structural trauma may create a cranial fault or cervical subluxation, interfering with any or all of these reflexes, causing considerable stress. This could result in suboccipital neuralgia and further cranial primary respiratory dysfunction with the potential for . . . health problems.

In simpler language, the head and neck can be bumped, as they often are, and the trauma, even minor, may cause processes for all kinds of faulty nerve signals that can trigger symptoms of severe conditions elsewhere in the body. Whether serious symptoms develop or not, chances are that the structural trauma contributes to some body disorganization, and the only way to tell is through the procedures of applied kinesiology.

My own case of hypoadrenia, caused primarily by habitual coffee drinking, serves as another good example of 'dietary imbalance or adverse environmental chemicals causing improper signaling of both the nervous and the endocrine systems,' as Dr Walther's text states. Insidious chemicals, often masquerading as harmless, abound in our environment. We hear *ad nauseam* about how our foods, our air and our water are loaded with them.

Causes for body disorganization from the structural and chemical sides of the triad of health are fairly easy to grasp. How the mental side of the triad relates to body organization is considerably more complex, and Dr Walther refers his students to research done by George B. Whatmore and Daniel R. Kohli, authors of *The Physiopathology and Treatment of Functional Disorders* (New York, 1974).

The two researchers theorize that several mechanisms, both mental and physical, create errors in nerve signaling. They call these garbled nerve signal mechanisms 'dysponesis', a word not yet in the dictionary that combines 'dys,' bad, faulty or wrong, with the root 'ponos,' meaning effort, work or toil. Dysponesis is, therefore, faulty effort. The researchers show that dysponesis can arise as a result of 'thought patterns which are not in the individual's best interest.' The negative thought patterns are not necessarily those familiar to everyone such as strong guilt feelings, bitter jealousy, unmitigated grief or violent hatred. These common psychological negatives do cause psychosomatic damage, but so do thought patterns of much lesser intensity, such as dwelling or overconcentrating on some small exterior stimulus — a minor itch, for example, or a scab covering a laceration. Studies have been conducted on the physiology or 'somato-automatic reflexes,' having to do with the powers of mind over parts of our bodies. Psychological stress can cause ulcers, for example. The same energy patterns created by the synapse mechanisms of our brains in the process of thinking can influence the energy patterns of autonomic nerve signals and thereby cause a physical manifestation of a mentally induced fault. Conversely, research in other areas indicates that one's mental attitude can assist the body when recovering from illness or trauma.

To improve a switched condition, or faulty body organization, applied kinesiologists have designed a series of simple exercises they call 'nerve patterning procedures.' Once the muscle-testing procedures determine the nature of body disorganization, the 'reeducation' of nerve signals can begin. The more disorganized the condition, the more difficult it is to do the exercises. However, one should perform the exercises as specifically instructed, otherwise the procedures will not only fail to help, but could worsen the condition. One should never ever give nerve patterning procedures to family or friends to try. Let them be examined, evaluated by muscle testing and given the pattern procedures suited to their particular body requirements.

The exercises are not designed to strengthen muscles, they are designed to educate nerve communication. Muscles will immediately get stronger when the procedures are done correctly; or weaker when they are performed incorrectly. The procedure will not 'cure' any disease or condition, but it will help the AK physician 'gain the most correction in the least amount of time and treatments.' It will also help prevent 'back-sliding,' on the part of the one being treated.

Dr Walther suggests the use of the 'cross crawl patterning', originally developed by two researchers who were seeking to treat speech and reading problems, and further developed by Dr Goodheart. The lying procedure is performed as follows:

Lying on back with legs straight and arms at sides, bring (right or left as instructed) arm and opposite leg up, bending at knee. Simultaneously turn head to the side of the raising arm, take a deep breath, and look up toward the raising arm.

Lower arm and leg, breathe out, and return head and eyes to neutral.

Bring opposite arm and leg up, bending at knee, keep head straight; simultaneously take a deep breath and look up toward the raising arm as the arm and leg come up.

Lower arm and leg, breathe out, and return eyes to neutral.

Dr Walther points out that this procedure represents one cycle and he suggests each doctor determine the number of cycles each patient should complete each day. Additionally, he advises to 'be certain to think through all of the processes as this is a mind-body procedure. Doing the pattern by habit is not very effective.'

For the standing move the procedure is explained as follows:

Standing, move right arm and opposite leg back as far as they will go. Simultaneously turn head to the same side as the arm that is going back, take a deep breath, and turn eyes toward the backward movement of the arm.

Bring arm, leg, head and eyes back to neutral and breathe out.

Next, bring opposite arm and leg back. Keep head straight; simultaneously take a deep breath and turn eyes toward the backward movement of the arm.

Bring arm, leg and eyes back to neutral and breathe out.

Once again there will be specific instructions on the number of these cycles to complete per day, and if you are instructed 'left' do them exactly the opposite of these examples.

I personally have not needed such nerve patterning procedures, but they were used to excellent effect by Sam, whose tennis game has remained strong and consistent since solving his switching.

There is still more that applied kinesiologists have incorporated into their practice in order to solve problems generally overlooked by other disciplines. Standard medical texts, for example, deal at length with the innate activities of body organization such as digestion, excretion, temperature control, acid-alkaline balance and so forth, and the AK physician studies all of it. However, he also studies in detail the 'inborn organization' that is not discussed in most standard tests. Here the applied kinesiologist is dealing with the dual-hemisphere brain and the phenomenon of 'unilateral brain function': While most of our nerve fibers cross over from left brain to right side and vice-versa, there are some that do not. The nerve patterns that do not cross over allow our bodies to adjust for operation of both sides of the body by one brain hemisphere in case of damage to the other hemisphere. Such brain damage prior to the age of four is usually compensated for readily, but by the time one is an adult damage to one hemisphere will generally impair specialized function.

Researchers have known about hemispherical specialization of the brain for more than a hundred years, and today it is generally understood that the left side of the brain is responsible for logic, precision, mathematics, accounting and factual data cataloging while the right side specializes in creativity, artistic forms, and imaginings. Most people tend to be dominant in one direction or the other — either logic or fancy, numbers or art. Of course, to be normal is to have a relative balance of both hemisphere influences so the dominance is not so strong as to cause maladjustment.

I'm left-handed, which means I'm not only in the minority in the worldwide population, but in certain circles I'm considered a little strange, or at least different. Left-handed persons make up only 5 percent of the population. The world in general, at least the manmade part of it, is right-hand-oriented in deference to the vast majority of people. Researchers have concluded that the right/left dominance is not only more prevalent, but it is an indication that right-handedness is a sign of more consistent development of the two sides of the brain. Regardless of which hemisphere is dominant, the normally functioning human brain features significant communication between its two sides. This communication occurs primarily through the corpus callosum behind the eyes (see Figure 23). This cross-brain communication

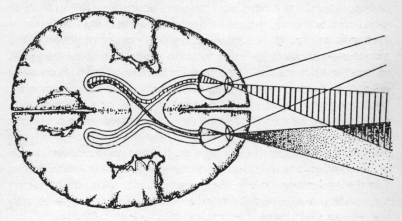

Figure 23. Corpus callosum.

is vital for optimum body function and organization. It has been discovered, incidentally, that animals do not have this same feature of laterality and interplay between the hemispheres of the brain: it is a phenomenon found only in humans.

Machines called electroencephalographs are used to reveal hemispheric brain function. These machines measure brain waves electronically. The living brain produces electromagnetic waves in specific frequencies. This bioelectrical activity has been the subject of considerable research in recent years. Our brains produce four distinct brain wave frequencies or patterns and these have been assigned Greek letter designators. When we are wide awake or fully conscious we are generally in the 'beta' state, which produces between 13.5 and 27 cycles of bioelectrical waves per second. As we relax or enter a meditative state our brainwaves slow down. The 'alpha' state is a conscious state, but one in which we are considerably relaxed. The alpha range is between 7 and 13.5 cycles, with the vast majority of meditative states registering 10.6 cycles. The 10.6-cycle brainwave rate for the vast majority of persons in a meditative state is interesting because it matches perfectly the 10.6 cycles of the resonance between our planet and its ionosphere, called Schumann resonances. Researchers have yet to hypothesize on the significance of that correlation. When we are asleep or unconscious our brain waves slow down to the 'theta' stage, which is between 3 and 7 cycles per second. The deepest sleep states are known as 'delta' states and the very slow cycles range between .02 and 3 cycles per second. Brainwave researchers have also tested the cycles produced from each separate brain hemisphere while subjects react to various stimuli. It was discovered that when a verbal test is administered the subjects usually experience alpha rhythm more on the right hemisphere than on the left. In a spatial test, the opposite is true. The conclusion is that there is a turning off of the information processing in the hemisphere registering the slower alpha cycles, thus allowing the opposite hemisphere to concentrate using fully conscious beta cycles.

Applied kinesiologists have a marked interest in some of the applications of this brainwave and body organization knowledge to specific body functions. While treating my hypoadrenia, Dr Hetrick guided me through some simple mental exercises, which I first thought of as rather silly. You may recall that I've already mentioned the muscle-testing procedure wherein he asked me to turn my head right and aim my eyes left and so forth. This time he asked me to simply count by fours.

'What?'

'Count by fours,' Dr Hetrick repeated as he cradled my leg in the position to test my sartorius.

I did as requested and naturally I had to concentrate to recall the correct sequence. As I concentrated on the count my muscle suddenly tested weak. This body language told Dr Hetrick that my adrenals needed still more therapy. The sudden weakening of the muscle after other forms of therapy had strengthened it told him that body disorganization was also involved in the glandular problem.

'Now, hum the tune to "Happy Birthday," ' he requested, again poised to test my leg muscle.

'Aw doc,' I protested, 'I can't carry a tune.'

'Just hum what you think to be the tune,' he insisted.

I rendered my tuneless rendition and he again tested the muscle. This time it tested strong, which indicated that the right hemisphere of my brain, the side responsible for creativity, was evidently not involved in the apparent body disorganization. It is interesting to note that the patient is asked to hum rather than sing the tune. Lyrics acquire 'verbal' activity, hence the realm of the left, not right, brain.

That there are practical applications for all this bilateral brain information tells us even more about the applied kinesiologist and the lengths to which this practitioner will go to better serve his patients. The ability to discern diagnostic information from our muscle reactions to left-brain/right-brain activity is simply part of the complexities AK physicians probe in order to be better doctors.

If you thought that perhaps the brain hemisphere dominance factors in therapy localization seemed a little gimmicky, wait until we've told you about the 'temporal tap.' The temporal tap, according to Dr Walther, 'is an applied kinesiologist's mechanism for penetrating the filter of the sensory system.' It is generally understood that there are certain body mechanisms that control our sensory abilities automatically. Our system is designed to filter, or otherwise appropriately deal with whatever stimuli our senses encounter. There is so much sensory activity bombarding our beings all the time that our bodies would be worn to a frazzle just sensing all of it. Since most of it is unnecessary for our survival, or our normal everyday functioning, our well-organized body systems filter most of it out for us.

Our eyes filter out most of the light spectrum, or else we would not be able to see very well. The clothing we wear contacts our body, but we are generally unaware of the touching sensations. When air conditioning is turned on, we may be acutely aware of the noise, the cooler air and the air movement, but within a short time our senses adapt to the change and filter out the sensations so we can get about our business.

Researchers also know that previous experience plays a role in our sense perceptions. If you have ever been drilled by a dentist and felt pain, you will not have the same sensory perception upon seeing and hearing the high speed dental equipment as a person would who had never experienced a modern dental office in his life. Our mental attitude, framed by our experiences, can modify the mechanisms that influence, or filter, our sensory processes.

The 'temporal tap seems to be a mechanism which provides an opportunity for working with these processes.' Dr Walther uses the 'seems to be' phrase because AK physicians are working more in the realm of hypothesis in temporal tapping than they are in hard-and-fast knowledge. Nevertheless, clinical results support the existing theory. Dr Walther, ever conservative as behooves the professional researcher, reminds his students that 'we must be careful about premature conclusions. The results of temporal tap are philosophically intriguing and seem to be clinically effective.'

The temporal tap came to Dr Goodheart's attention when he read some fascinating reports by a Czechoslovakian doctor who allegedly helped persons reduce smoking by giving them positive affirmations while manipulating the temporal bone, which is the bone on the side of the head, above and in front of each ear. The Czech physician died before Goodheart could contact him, but the founder of applied kinesiology decided to experiment with penetrating the sensory system by transmitting positive and negative thoughts, and other stimuli, while manipulating the temporal bone. At first he was unsuccessful, but after considerable experience, he found success.

Applied kinesiologists are taught temporal tapping from a diagram outlining the temporal sphenoidal (TS) diagnostic line (see Figure 24). The ear cavity and temporomandibular joint (TMJ) are just below the TS line.

Like palpating or other aspects of a manipulative physician's practice, temporal tapping is a highly skilled procedure, and its proper use can be yet another diagnostic tool for isolating and ferreting out basic causes of a particular symptom. Walther says 'the temporal tap is used to penetrate the sensory filter, influence some types of therapy, control some involuntary activities, and give additional therapy localization information.' However, the physician must have already determined the patient's brain hemisphere dominance, or whether the patient is a mixed dominance type, before applying temporal tap procedure.

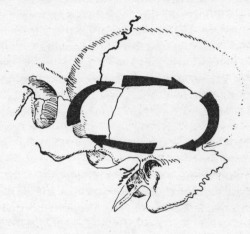

Figure 24.   The temporal sphenoidal diagnostic line.

Correct temporal tapping always begins just in front of the ear and progresses clockwise around the TS line. The tapping should be crisp enough to make the physician's fingers bounce away from the skull after each tap, but should not be so hard that the patient feels pain. Dr Walther says that other methods of stimulating the TS line have been tried, such as ultrasound, vibrators, pinching, rubbing and electrical stimulation, but they have not demonstrated any effectiveness.

I asked Dr Hetrick if he tapped the left side of my head because I was left-brain dominant. 'No,' he replied, 'I tap everyone on the left side except in very specific instances.' His response ruined a theory I was forming about this strange new subject. Evidently my facial expression told him I was trying to form new questions, so he volunteered answers on the spot.

'Temporal tapping seems to reach a more subtle level of the nervous system. I use it primarily to determine if more work needs to be done. For example, we've been working on your lymphatic reflexes and it's time to determine if the therapy has been sufficient or more needs to be done. You might require chemical support, and the temporal tap will improve the chemical support indicators, which will take the form of additional muscle tests.'

Almost as an aside, Dr Hetrick recalled the circumstances of Dr Goodheart's discovery of the temporal tap phenomenon. 'I've found that I can use the temporal tap for conditioning,' he added. 'For example, if a patient has a gag reflex and I'm going to make cranial adjustments with my fingers inside his mouth, I'll temporal tap on the left side of his head and make a positive suggestion that he doesn't need to gag, and it will work. For conditioning I tap the left side for positive input and the right side for a negative input.'

If we patients choose to remain skeptical, we might look at it this way: temporal tapping doesn't hurt, it doesn't raise the doctor's fees, and it may provide additional information about a condition that may otherwise be overlooked. However, if your AK physician wants to add a fat surcharge to his fee for tapping your temporal, I'd suggest holding off for more research. At this time, temporal tapping seems to be an excellent 'audit mechanism' that applied kinesiologists may use to determine whether all of the five systems have been fully explored and possibly corrected. Those five systems, again, include the nervous system, circulatory system, lymphatic system, skeletal-musculature system and the acupuncture meridians.

Chapter Nine:

Nutrition, Polarity and Ongoing Research

Many times we have heard the expression 'You are what you eat' from persons who advocate diets that are more natural. However, research has shown that truth may be better served if the adage were to be 'You are what you metabolize.' Civilized human beings eat a tremendous variety of foods and non foods, and vitamin supplements. Perhaps it is a good thing that very little of it is actually metabolized and used in body functions. Applied kinesiology offers a useful tool for physicians to determine a patient's actual nutritional needs and metabolic status. Muscle testing does not take the place of careful laboratory analyses of blood and other diagnostic testing, but it is an outstanding adjunct to what other diagnostic tests may tell the physician. Drs Goodheart, Walther and Hetrick all stress that AK muscle-testing procedures are primarily a means of obtaining more information about individual nutritional needs, and should not be used as the only source of that information.

Your body's reaction to a particular foodstuff or supplement may be tested by AK procedures. Continuing research is making this medical art more of a clinical science with each passing year. In time, it may be proved that the muscle-testing procedures related to nutrition and metabolism are, indeed, infallible or extremely accurate, but until that time, experimentation is ongoing — and fascinating.

We have seen demonstrations by persons claiming an ability to 'dowse' food or nutritional supplements with a pendulum dangling from their fingers. If the pendulum swings clockwise, the dowsers claim, the substance is 'good for you,' and if the pendulum rotates counter-clockwise, it is 'negative.' The accuracy of such dowsing is subject to a great deal of skepticism, but the idea that polarity exists is the substance of scientific research.

Body metabolism is what we do with all the food, water and air we take into our systems. Through metabolism that incoming material is converted into energy and growth and repair and waste to be eliminated. Scientists have learned the most about metabolism from studying the blood. Our vascular system carries all the nutrients to all the cells throughout our body, and carries away the waste products of each cell. Reading and analyzing blood chemistry has taught us a great deal. AK physicians are taught to use muscle testing to supplement and double-check blood and urine test information. Over the years it developed that muscle testing, especially the series of tests involving leg 'turn-in,' which is associated with walking movement called 'gait mechanism,' has particular value in helping AK physicians gauge metabolism effects. It has been hypothesized that the gait mechanism affects body energy patterns in such a way as to affect metabolism, and conversely, that metabolism may affect the gait mechanism.

According to Dr Hetrick, 'We are taught that riboflavin and niacin . . . contribute to the relative polarity of red blood cells.' The term 'polarity' deals with more than surface charge, considering other energy factors. 'It's been established with reasonable certainty that the red blood cells have a positive polarity,' Dr Hetrick explained. 'The arterial wall, and the venous wall, the white blood cells and blood platelets all have a positive polarity, so they all repel each other. This prevents them from clogging together or sludging the blood.'

The body has ways of recognizing polarity instantly, and the body's polarity detection mechanisms are considerably more effective than the most massive equipment we have designed and built.

Recent experiments have shown that AK muscle testing indicates that a method of chemically assaying the blood is incomplete and AK procedures provide more complete data. According to Dr Goodheart, George Miroff, who heads the Monroe Medical Laboratory in Monroe, New York, described at one of Dr

Goodheart's seminars some studies carried out with a large number of schizophrenics, people suffering from a mental disorder commonly called 'split personality.' Some psychiatric researchers today have been treating schizophrenia with massive doses of vitamins in a procedure called orthomolecular therapy. Dr Miroff's study found that although only 3 percent of the schizophrenics showed any deficiencies of nutrients in their bloodstreams, when they were treated with the megadoses of orthomolecular nutrition, a staggering 70 percent responded.

Obviously, the method used to analyze the patients' blood in this study had not revealed essential data, but under those conditions, Dr Miroff developed the functional assays for the nutritional approach to schizophrenia. In describing Dr Miroff's work, Dr Goodheart pointed out that applied kinesiology provides as good a 'functional assay' as can be imagined. He explained his point of view with the following analogy:

> When you measure the bloodstream nutrients in a laboratory test tube, you are measuring what is in the transport system. In other words, your check is in the mail, but you can't put that in the bank until you actually get it. The transport system cannot measure the use system. You may have a chiropractic office, and tables and secretaries and so forth, but the use of it is how many patients you treat.

Dr Miroff showed that the functional assays of the schizophrenic cases indicated a much higher percentage of deficiency than the 3 percent indicated by lab analysis of the bloodstream.

Dr Miroff's findings were paralleled by AK researchers in a study of 25 cases of carpal tunnel syndrome (painful problems with a wrist joint) wherein all 25 patients were scheduled for corrective surgery. Prior to surgery, all 25 patients were given doses of 1250 milligrams of vitamins B_6. The patients' blood was analyzed by laboratory methods and the serum indicated that the level of B_6 was better than normal; that there was adequate B_6 available in the transport system. However, when the level of B_6 was measured within the red cell, it was deficient. More B_6 was given and eventually all 25 patients improved and did not require surgery. Dr Goodheart said, 'The lesson here is plain — the body can maintain the B_6 level normal in serum, yet it can be low in the red cells.' Other nutritional researchers such as William Donald Kelley, the founder of computerized metabolic typing for individuals, have shown that in a vast number of individuals metabolic absorption of specific nutrients is faulty. Dr Kelley has shown that if an 'ordinary' dose of vitamins does not seem to affect a particular symptom, in many cases much larger doses will eventually have a proportionate absorption to the correct level of function. The B_6 example further confirms this fact of nutritional and metabolic life.

Why does absorption failure occur? Why does the metabolism appear to go only partway with some nutrients? Dr Goodheart pointed out that although 70 percent of the schizophrenic patients improved with megavitamin, orthomolecular therapy, 30 percent did not. Why not? 'Despite the fact they [the patients] were getting the equivalent of 30 pounds of honey and 50 pounds of beefsteak, the 30 percent didn't respond,' Dr Goodheart stressed. 'They tried the intramuscular and the I.V. routes, and only about 3 percent of the people improved — which meant there was some other factor.'

Dr Goodheart then reasoned that the 'red cells were positive, the blood vessel wall was positive, the platelets were positive, the white cells were positive, and that for anything to enter across the brush border membrane of the small intestine it would either have to be negative or less positive than those materials that are in the bloodstream.'

The innovative Dr Goodheart then conducted tests on patients with gait problems and without gait problems. You may recall that gait, the walking or running motion, requires body organization, and that disorganization in the body may affect many aspects of body function. Using AK muscle-testing procedures and standard uncoated nutrient tablets placed on patients' tongues, with several variations, Dr Goodheart made a discovery. He learned that 'tongue placement in terms of the tablet was important.'

The patients were muscle-tested with a tablet containing

necessary nutrients placed on the center of the tongue; with the tablet position reversed but still placed on the center of the tongue; with the tablet placed on the left side of the tongue and moved forward and backward along the tongue. All produced similar positive response in the test muscle. However, testing the tablet on the right side of the tongue in many patients had no effect. Dr Goodheart mused: 'Is it possible that the foot is the generator-alternator and the brain is the battery, with the spinal cord and nerves all the electrical connections? Perhaps the body is the fan, and there may be a loose fan belt somewhere. The hip joint on one side is like an old-fashioned static generator or an old-fashioned telephone where you had to crank it to generate current.'

Dr Goodheart then carried his electrical analogy further in order to offer possible insight into the phenomenon of polarity and its possible effect on nutrient metabolism. 'I wondered if it were possible that one side cranks positive and the other side cranks negative and that polarity differences can be altered. In other words, the right side of the body is positive on the anterior and negative on the posterior; the left side of the body is negative on the anterior and positive on the posterior.'

If such circuitry could be firmly established, a reason for the failure of certain individuals to absorb nutrients that are available in the bloodstreams and get those nutrients on the job at their functional station would be established. From that point, it would be merely a matter of additional muscle-testing procedures and therapy localizations to locate the part of a patient's body, probably the hip joints if Dr Goodheart is correct in his theory, that are short-circuiting the polarity mechanism.

The late Albert Roy Davis, Ph.D., of Green Cove Springs, Florida, was the world's leading researcher into biomagnetism, the study of magnetic influences on biological organisms. Established medical science has not yet shown any serious interest in Davis's lifelong research, but Dr Goodheart and others who have encountered the complex mechanisms of polarity in its various energy forms have found Davis's work extremely interesting.

Quite by accident back in the early 1930s, the young physicist discovered that the energy emitted from the poles of a magnet was not the same. The south pole magnetism is different from the north pole magnetism. This is still not generally accepted in scientific circles, but Davis proved the difference thousands of times in experiments with living organisms. Manmade machines and apparatus might not be able to detect the difference between south pole magnetism and north pole magnetism, but biological organisms can. The accident that opened this unique area of research to Davis featured two cartons of earthworms that Davis had set on his work bench in anticipation of a fishing trip the following day. Also resting on that bench was a large horseshoe magnet. The worms, in thin cardboard containers, were placed near the two poles of the magnet, virtually in the magnetic fields emanating from the strong permanent magnet's open ends. The container next to the south pole was eaten through by the agitated and active worms, but those in the other container simply lay around inside as worms generally do. Davis deduced that the south pole of the strong magnet must have somehow affected the worms.

Later experiments proved the vast differences between the two magnetic poles and the consistent effects such magnetism can have on living biological organisms. To prove the thesis of his discovery, Davis began a series of experiments that continued the rest of his life. Subsequent research proved that south magnetic polarity stimulated remarkable increases in animal energies, growth and disposition. Chicks hatched under the influence of south magnetic polarity, for example, grew to be larger, meaner and more ferocious roosters, and this result was invariable. North magnetic polarity, however, has the opposite effect on hatching chickens. North pole magnetism made wimps of the maturing chicks — invariably. Chickens hatched and raised under influences of both magnetic polarities were 'normal.'

Using the separate and distinct magnetic polarities, Davis and his associate Walter Rawls designed and built equipment for stimulating the germination of seeds and the improvement of crop yields and resistance to disease and drought. Davis also spent decades in studying the use of the two distinct polarities in the promotion of healing human disease. Health practitioners had been using magnets in various and sundry ways throughout much of history, but Davis proved that indiscriminate use of magnetic energy in attempts at healing was unwise. Davis explained some of his research this way:

> We have dissolved calcium in animal joints that is equivalent to arthritis in humans; we have controlled pain in blood-circulating animals, which we believe is an important discovery that medical researchers should study further. We have found that the north pole of a magnet can arrest and control certain types of cancers as well as reduce swellings and infections. North pole energy has extended the normal life spans of small animals up to 50 percent.

Davis also pointed out that one would not use the south pole magnetism in treating certain cancers because the malignancy would be enhanced by south pole energy. Throughout his lifetime, Davis constantly sought recognition and peer review for his biomagnetic research, but none was forthcoming. His books, written with Rawls, include *The Magnetic Effect* and *Magnetism and Its Effect on the Living System,* and they may be purchased from Associated Partners West, P.O. Box 641, Solana Beach, California 92075. They are not generally available in bookstores.

Continuing the exploration of polarity, metabolism and body energy patterns, Dr Goodheart stresses that since the poles of a magnet are opposite forms of the magnetic energy, and living organisms understand that subtle difference and may be affected by it, then if food or nutrients have different polarity qualities (as dowsers claim to demonstrate), it is feasible that if the digestive gradient is disturbed by too much positive polarity on one side and not enough on the other, balance will be disturbed.

'The only place you can really, non-invasively, observe the digestive tract in terms of its potential polarity might be the tongue,' Goodheart suggests. 'Could that be the reason why we have alterations in the saliva flow on one side or the other? Is that why teeth can sometimes decay on one side of the mouth and not on the other? Is that the reason why one would occasionally get a disturbance on the one side and not the other?'

AK researchers continue exploring the parallels between gait mechanism and potential polarity imbalances in the digestive tract. Recalling the key difference between 'transport' and 'use' of nutrients by the bloodstream, Dr Goodheart expounds:

> For example, if you have a polarity difference on the right side of your small intestine and it has the wrong polarity, you won't get the absorption needed and you might have to push 10 times as much nutrition past there to get one-tenth the amount of absorption. Then, further along the intestine, the polarity might have a different pattern, but that one side being disturbed would make the other side disturbed as well. . ..
>
> I can remember doing neurolymphatic activity [stimulating a patient's lymphatic system by vigorously massaging a particular point on the patient's body associated with the portion of the lymphatic system the physician desires to stimulate — in this patient's case, massaging on his liver].
>
> . . . Later the patient told me his night blindness problem was stopped without the addition of vitamin A. Frequently, structural corrections were accomplished which corrected specific vitamin B disorders — disorders that I could measure, and which appeared to be nutritional. Now we can see a reason for it. Certainly for the night blindness, I didn't add any vitamin A, and by the same token, making structural corrections in the pelvis must alter the availability of nutrients. One can be aware of the fact that it happened, but not aware of how it was accomplished.

Dr Goodheart is certain that structural corrections will influence cell metabolism, bionic activity and balances in the body's electron poising (pronounced *pwazing*) system, which is a physiological system for controlling the viscosity of fluids and the dynamics of velocity within those fluids — a complicated phenomenon of physics discovered and measured by a French physician named Jean Louis Marie Poiseuille.

In my own case, I have learned that my body fails to absorb

a great deal of the expensive vitamin, mineral and glandular extract supplementation I've been taking. My pelvis has been 'rotated' and imbalanced for many years and it has taken a lot of work by Dr Hetrick to get my structure back in place and to have it stay there. Dr Goodheart's research is not yet conclusive, but enough has been demonstrated to make his theories credible.

If you'd like to have some fun, create some bumper stickers that read: 'Wobbly hips mean lousy nutrition,' or 'better femural angulation for better night vision.' Not only would those bumper stickers cause some head scratching, they could be true.

Dr Goodheart summed up his studies of polarity, nutrition and the probable gait mechanism connection somewhat philosophically as follows:

A necessary corollary would be for us to try to understand what the positivity and negativity of foods may be. I am sure oriental ideas (yin and yang — acupuncture) make sense. It makes much more sense to organize the body and let the body choose from an ample and wide spectrum diet rather than continually reducing the dietary pattern. We are surrounded by nutrients, and it never did make sense that some nutrients should be unnatural or bad for you, or worse than others. It certainly makes much more sense that the body is rejecting it rather than the food itself is inimical to man's metabolism.

When the food is altered by man [refined, hydrogenated, pasteurized, homogenized, chemicalized *ad nauseam*]; altered in its constituency and its oxidation potential [such as listed above], that is another matter. However, to continually reduce the foods that apparently seem to interfere or disagree with someone is to reduce an already poor diet, and I think that particular concept is wrong. It would seem to me that one should be able to eat a Coney Island hot dog or some other thing that isn't good for you, without getting sick. If you get sick every time from eating relatively good food, I don't think it means the food is wrong, it means that something in you is wrong. Someone should investigate you rather than making the concerted effort to do cytotoxic testing [cell testing for allergy], which is a good idea, but somewhat subject to error. It would be much more reasonable to fix the body rather than to alter the diet. This relatively simple observation goes a long way toward understanding nutrition. Therefore, to get optimum uptake, we should have optimum physical health and optimum physical balance, and balancing the structure is one way to obtain it.

If Dr Goodheart is right about that, it means I will be able to drink coffee with cream and sugar without suffering any ill effects once my structure is completely corrected, and all the deleterious effects on my glands and organs have been corrected. Sounds too good to be true, but I can hope. The biggest problem I have, and many patients like me will have, is that a deleterious habit continues during treatment, helping make it more difficult for the physician to get me back into near-perfect condition.

Applied kinesiology has demonstrated, time and again, that the human body is a totally integrated network of complex systems, and often something as simple as 'thin-air' can have an effect on a particular aspect of one system and thereby wind up affecting the overall. For example, there is the research into what have come to be called 'electro dermal points' — which correspond to acupuncture points. (To demonstrate the connection, a researcher took a portable electronic unit that had a long wire lead with a tiny light bulb attached to a metal probe on the end, and he glided the probe across my naked torso. Whenever the probe met an acupuncture juncture, the light shone. Not surprisingly, the modern electronic probe confirmed the ancient acupuncture points.)

Dr Goodheart tells of a Hungarian researcher who measured the amount of carbon dioxide emitted from the body at the electro dermal point. The idea behind this particular research was to show that the acupuncture points were, indeed, a source of energy flow, even if that energy were merely an exchange of respiratory gas. We humans breathe through the pores of our skin, taking in oxygen and emitting carbon dioxide, just as we do with our lungs, only not at anything near the same volume and scale.

Applied kinesiologists have experimented by taking the fact

of skin respiration a step further and observing muscle reactions with known AK testing procedures. Under certain conditions, it was discovered, placing carbon dioxide gas (found in soft drinks everywhere) on the skin would cause a detectable weakness of certain body patterns. The observed weaknesses could then be neutralized or strengthened by oxygen. Conversely, the AK probers would surround portions of the skin with pure oxygen to weaken or neutralize certain energy patterns that had been enhanced by applications of carbon dioxide. That our bodies have definite reactions to the content of atmospheric gases should not be surprising. City dwellers, in particular, are walking around in a sea of carbon dioxide, oxygen, nitrogen and a myriad of pollutants all the time, and the physical effects of the condition of the air in numerous cities are well known. Los Angeles has its famous 'smog alerts', called when the air is so polluted that it is said to be 'unhealthful for all persons.' A less serious 'alert' tells us that the air is 'unhealthful for the very old, or the very young and persons with respiratory problems.' The smog conditions are broadcast daily. AK researchers have begun investigating the influence of common gases on our skins.

Dr Goodheart notes, 'It is surprising to see that carbon dioxide occasionally neutralizes the weakness that oxygen produces, and I was even more surprised to find oxygen weakening some patients. I knew that something was going on, but I didn't know exactly how to classify that particular situation. It seemed much more reasonable that oxygen should help, after all there is the accepted idea of hyperbaric oxygen and its relative use with some patients.' (Hyperbaric chambers are pressurized oxygen chambers which are used for specific kinds of patients by established medical practitioners.)

Goodheart continues: 'It is reasonable to assume that oxygen is of some value. Yet, there was solid evidence that on a large number of patients, oxygen's neutralizing effect seemed to be about equally divided, and I had trouble understanding that.'

Wouldn't the doctors using hyperbaric oxygen chambers be surprised, too?

To understand further what AK researchers are seeking to prove relative to the effects of carbon dioxide and oxygen contacting the surface of our skin, we need to somehow visualize the work of neurotransmitters, which are tiny packets of electrochemical data banks constantly relaying information to appropriate centers in our bodies. The evidence shows that the contact of carbon dioxide or oxygen gases to particular parts of our skin will affect the acupuncture points and subsequently will affect neurotransmitters. It is analogous to the foot muscle proprioceptors' sending faulty messages to other parts of the body and creating minor havoc until a symptom erupts. AK researchers are studying the possible relationship of a body's oxidation rate, an aspect of metabolism which varies from individual to individual, and the effects of carbon dioxide and/or oxygen on certain electro dermal points, such as those points located around the edge of your forefinger and thumb when you cup your hand.

One patient, known to be an overoxidizer, had been tested for the presence of carpal tunnel syndrome (a painful wrist joint problem). This patient was asked to breathe out on his hand area several times, bathing the hand in carbon dioxide. The exhaled carbon dioxide caused an immediate weakening of the test muscles. However, tests of the patient's respiratory system revealed no oxygen deficit. Another patient, known to be an underoxidizer, and also having carpal tunnel syndrome, did not weaken the test muscles by breathing his own carbon dioxide onto his hand area.

It was suggested that the first patient breathe his carbon dioxide on the second patient. It was done, but it didn't matter, the muscles did not weaken. However, when oxygen was sprayed on the second patient's hand, the muscles weakened. The second patient was tested for a respiratory oxygen deficit, and was demonstrated to be deficient.

Utilizing the 'electron poising curve,' Goodheart explained the latter experimental reactions. The electron poising curve is technical language for a curve or pattern demonstrating the connection between left-brain/right-brain activity and particular nutrients. AK researchers have learned that water-soluble vitamins trigger left-brain activity and fat-soluble vitamins trigger right-brain activity. Since correct body organization requires left-brain activity to affect right-sided muscles and vice versa, manual muscle-testing procedures will be accurate and effective tools only when specific nutrients and vitamins are tested on the proper sides. Water-soluble vitamin C, manganese and thyroid extract are listed as left-brain, right-sided muscle nutrients by the electron poising curve; fat-soluble vitamin E, zinc and adrenal or ovary extract are listed as right-brain, left-sided nutrients. Common to both sides are vitamin A, iron, copper and folic acid.

With these distinctions diagrammed on a chart, Dr Goodheart explains the oxygen-carbon dioxide experiments as follows:

> In a general sense, you can classify people on the electron poising curve. If you look at the chart, those to the left of the curve on the adrenal side will weaken dramatically with carbon dioxide, yet there is no sign that they need oxygen if you test them for oxygen deficit. Conversely, on the other end of the curve, the upper end, those individuals will not weaken from carbon dioxide, but will weaken from oxygen.

What we have here is a tool for evaluating a patient's metabolic oxidation rate — an evaluation that can be made on the spot with a living, breathing entity, and an evaluation that can be used to confirm or support laboratory information. Dr Goodheart notes that his research into the nutritional aspects of the various oxidizing capacities as reflected by his electron poising curve and the effects of carbon dioxide or oxygen, matches the conclusions and classifications produced by Dr George Watson, a noted researcher who is credited with establishing oxidation rate variables in people. Because people are biochemically individualized within a spectrum of a dozen basic metabolic types, any tool that helps the physician understand your particular individuality is valuable.

That a breath of carbon dioxide, or oxygen can actually strengthen muscles in some people under certain conditions led Goodheart to relate his personal observations of professional tennis players.

I was struck by the fact that if you watch world class tennis professionals, whether they are right hand or left handed, many times just before they serve they will cup their handed and breathe on it. [Strengthening the muscles? Instinctively?] I found that Connors or Lendl or Bjorg, or any of the tennis players who cupped their hand and breathed on it, did so consistently — but they would not do it in the fifth set of a hotly contested match!

Why not? Are we getting into numerology with the fifth set? No; Dr Goodheart offers a rationale:

As you go down past the center of the electron poising curve [categorizing individuals] you get into the stress pattern of the adrenal. The adrenal is a stress gland, and as you get further into the stress pattern you actually need something to relieve the stress. As the player breathes on his hand, it takes the tension down and out, and allows him to have more touch or control of the racquet. Still, in the fifth set, they didn't do it. I also observed that when it was a three set match, a player who breathed on his hand would do so if he was ahead of the other player by a large number of games, but if the contest were close, or if he was behind, he did not do it.

Perhaps there is a relay of body information going on within certain, highly skilled and highly trained tennis players who have worked hard to control their 'body organization' for better athletic performance, and some of these players react to this information by unconsciously blowing carbon dioxide on the key acupuncture points exposed by a cupped hand. When the body information reaches a 'hopeless' level of stress, the unconscious drive to blow on the hand simply isn't there.

Dr Goodheart's observations are interesting and provocative, and there may come a day when he applies that information to clinical research. Applied kinesiology is still a struggling new medical science with considerable promise for the future. Muscle-testing procedures are an effective way for determining individual physiological responses and reactions to just about any internal or external stimuli. The growing body of knowledge within applied kinesiology will one day be considered invaluable to medical diagnostics.

Chapter Ten:

How to Choose an AK Physician

Just because a person puts some letters after his name, hangs a sign up outside his office, makes his premises smell antiseptic, wears a white smock, and displays an official-looking piece of paper on his wall, does not mean he's a competent AK physician.

Of course, it's possible to have all those markings of the professional and be a quack, but that's generally not the case. Cynics feel that the most credentialed are often quacks of the highest magnitude. A credentialed quack is still a quack.

You can quickly distinguish between the competent practitioner and the quack by knowing what the AK physician has to offer. The practising AK is a graduate chiropractor who can explain to you how your glands and organs appear to be functioning with specific muscle tests. He can suggest nutrition to help improve various conditions, and he can demonstrate with your muscles that you probably need particular nutrients. He can correct problems in your spine and in joints, and can stretch or compress muscles to improve your structural condition. He may massage certain junctures of nerve, lymph, blood and acupuncture meridians to stimulate glandular or systemic activity. He can advise you on how to stay healthy and he will pay particular attention to your posture and your feet. He can offer an excellent second opinion if you are under a physician's care, are seeing a chiropractor who is not an applied kinesiologist, or if you have been in an accident. We have already discussed how helpful AK muscle testing can be following injury or trauma to the body.

But the AK physician cannot cure cancer or arthritis or diabetes. He cannot adjust you to overcome heart disease or stop the spread of infection. Applied kinesiology is not designed for crisis medicine. It is designed to be part of a holistic approach to preventive medicine. Don't forget this — and don't let him forget it either.

Judging competency is something we all must learn to do, and must try to practice all the time. Competent people know their business, and also their limitations. A competent applied kinesiologist can generally be judged best on the basis of what he knows and the limitations he admits.

Carole and I attended a health convention a few years ago, and one of the attractions on the showroom floor that caught our attention was a booth advertising 'pyramid power' among other things. The proprietor was selling 'pyramid energy' and some nutritional supplements that somehow enhanced one's sex life and energy when taken in conjunction with emanations from a model of the Great Pyramid in Egypt. The upshot of the sales pitch was a demonstration of pyramid-powered pills' having beneficial effect, which he 'proved' by placing the pill in a potential customer's mouth and using what was purported to be AK muscle-testing procedure.

He asked the eager guinea pigs, who lined up for the demo with wide-eyed, sometimes bemused, wonder, to extend their right arms out full-length and parallel to the floor. He then placed a pill in each mouth — alleging that it was 'ordinary' multiple vitamin in content, or words to that effect — his inconsistency tipped us off to his potential quackery. With the pill in the volunteer's mouth, the arm was easily pulled down by the peddler, who grinned as he demonstrated the muscle weakness. It was probably a sugar pill and as such would make nearly every person test weak in this manner, which is only a partial AK procedure. Predictably, after he plucked a pill from within the pyramid-shaped framework of his small model and placed it on the willing tongue, the same muscle tested 'strong.'

Not only was the muscle-testing procedure being used for the demonstration improper since the quack did not take pains to prevent a series of muscles from being involved rather than a single muscle, but there was no adequate demonstration that the pills he used for the 'weak' demonstration were in fact the same substance as those he plucked from his pyramid.

If this kind of chicanery goes on openly at 'health' conventions what might one encounter inside an office with a diploma framed and on the wall?

Several different times during my sessions with Dr Hetrick, he tested me for particular nutritional needs. In each case, he was painstakingly thorough, taking the time and energy to run through a complete series of therapy localizations on the particular aspect of my systems he was testing. It was hard work, and time-consuming — neither of which are advantageous to quackery. Of course, my intrinsic nature caused me to tease him, something like this: 'You must be short of cash, hey Doc? Whenever you need a few dollars extra, you test for nutrition needs and sell a bottle of snake oil, right?'

Although that sounds mean, it was taken with the humor intended. The competent AK physician can handle skepticism and cynicism, and his demonstrations of muscle-testing procedure can be repeated for you, right on the spot. Of course, you can be wasting valuable time he must subtract from other patients, so he may suggest increasing his fee to accommodate your chronic skepticism. It's a two-way street. Good doctors don't mind serious, probing questions from patients. You have a right to understand, and competent physicians will explain and demonstrate so that you can.

Suppose you are being tested for nutritional need and the AK physician places the tablet on your chest instead of on your tongue? Unfortunately, this has become standard practice in California, despite clear warnings from the International College of Applied Kinesiology (ICAK) that such procedures are not necessarily valid. Dr Hetrick, however, stayed within guidelines and tested for nutritional need by placing tablets on the patient's tongue only. Many others, we learned, simply place the tablet on the solar plexus, in front of the diaphragm, and then muscle-test for responses. They are accepting a school of thought that suggests the body detects the 'energy patterns' of the substance from the spot on the chest just as well as it does from the tongue. The method has also been used by some AK specialists to inform patients that they had allergies to certain foods. It's possible that the procedure might somehow be reliable, but a controlled study, conducted for the ICAK by John J. Triano demonstrated only a 'random' response in the use of muscle testing for nutrition needs, especially when the subject is not chewing or tasting the substance being evaluated.

The executive board of the International College of Applied Kinesiology on 23 May 1983, issued an 'adopted status statement,' which provides a clear picture of what you can expect from a competent AK physician. Some of this will seem repetitious at this point, but on the other hand, you should have no trouble understanding it now:

> The use of manual muscle testing to evaluate body function as introduced by George J. Goodheart, Jr., D.C., in 1964 has provided an additional dimension to the diagnosis of human dysfunction. The initial protocol of examination was limited to the evaluation and improvement of structural balance.
>
> Early in its development it became obvious that many of the treatment methods used in chiropractic and other disciplines of the healing arts improved muscle function as perceived by manual muscle testing. Standard therapeutic approaches make up the majority of treatment techniques developed which are unique to applied kinesiology.
>
> The most important value of applied kinesiology is its ability as a system of evaluating function to give added dimension to diagnosis. The manual muscle test does not evaluate the strength a muscle can generate; rather, it evaluates the ability of the body's controlling system, for example, the nervous system, to adapt the muscle to meet the changing pressure of the examiner's test. This requires that the examiner be well-trained in the anatomy and physiology of muscle function. The action of the muscle being tested, as well as how the body recruits synergistic muscles, must be known. Manual muscle testing is a science and an art, with emphasis on the science.
>
> Many unique observations have been made in applied kinesiology which have given a better insight into body function. It is the ICAK's position that applied kinesiology examination

should be combined with standard physical diagnosis, laboratory, x-ray, history, and any other special examination procedures of the physician who is using applied kinesiology as an adjunct to diagnosis. AK examination should *enhance standard diagnosis, not replace it* [emphasis added].

Applied kinesiology methods add information to an examination, but they should not be used as the major investigative endeavor. These procedures — such as therapy localization, nutritional testing, establishing dental vertical dimension, the muscle/organ association, etc. — can help the physician determine the major cause of a patient's health problem. They should be used with other supporting evidence from standard techniques in diagnosis. Rarely, if ever, should a diagnosis be made on limited and restricted examination. A limited approach, whatever the method, can lead to error.

Therapy localization is a phenomenon for which the current data base of knowledge has no adequate explanation. Efforts have been and are being made to better understand the mechanism. When positive therapy localization is present, other examination findings should be used to determine, and finally confirm, the diagnosis. For example, positive therapy localization to a vertebral area requires further examination by palpation of the intrinsic muscles, motion palpation, x-ray (if needed), vertebral challenge, and the structures innervated by the area. Finally, when all factors are considered and a subluxation or fixation is diagnosed and adjusted, therapy localization — as well as other findings — gives the physician feedback as to whether the corrective effort was successful.

Nutritional evaluation should be done only with the subject chewing the substance. It is also necessary to evaluate other factors which may influence the perceived muscle strength. Confirming diagnostic criteria for the need of any nutrition should be present from the patient's other diagnostic work-up, which may include history, type of dysfunction, laboratory tests, physical diagnosis, and dietary inadequacies.

The ICAK specifically does not approve of the use of manual muscle testing as a single method in determining an individual's nutritional needs. Research sponsored by the ICAK revealed a random response to blind testing of nutrition when the latissimus dorsi muscle was tested. Further research is under way to put into perspective the change perceived in manual muscle testing when nutrition is tested.

The use of manual muscle testing to evaluate nutrition is particularly a problem when done by lay nutrition sales persons as a tool to sell their product. Not only should a person have an educational background to evaluate nutritional needs; the use of manual muscle testing requires a high level of knowledge in the proper muscle testing techniques.

The muscle/organ association used in applied kinesiology is referred to as 'body language.' A close clinical association has been observed between specific muscle dysfunction and related organ or gland dysfunction. This has never been considered an absolute in applied kinesiology. It gives the physician an indication of the organs or glands to consider as possible sources of health problems. In standard diagnosis, body language is seen in many anemic individuals as paleness, fatigue, and lack of color in the capillaries and arterioles of the internal surface of the lower eyelid, giving the physician an indication that anemia may be present. An actual diagnosis of anemia is not justified without a blood count. The same type of body language indications comes from the muscle-gland-organ consideration in applied kinesiology. Further examination may or may not confirm an association in the particular case being studied. It is the physician's total diagnostic work-up which determines the final diagnosis.

Unfortunately, there are those — both lay persons and professionals who use manual muscle testing without the necessary expertise. There are others who fail to co-ordinate the AK findings with other standard diagnostic procedures. This lack of knowledge or correlation of findings may cause erroneous interpretation of the condition present and lead to improper treatment, or failure to treat the appropriate condition.

When placed in proper perspective, applied kinesiology is indeed adding a new dimension to diagnosis. It is valuable primarily in functional conditions. It helps the physician to understand the symptomatic complexes which are not pathological in nature, as well as why pathology has developed.

The proper use of applied kinesiology requires an appreciation and understanding of anatomy and physiology. The physician must have an excellent understanding of muscular synergism to be able to properly administer manual muscle testing.

Of course, we must realize that the ICAK is an institutional body and is therefore subject to a certain conservatism. Most likely, the actual truth of the value of applied kinesiology lies beyond even some of the seemingly improbable relationships only touched upon in this book.

Dr Hetrick serves as a model of professional protocol for AK physicians. For example, he asked me to stick a thermometer under my arm and measure my temperature every morning before getting out of bed for a period of ten days, merely to substantiate what his muscle-testing procedures had told him about my potential for hyperthyroidism. He really didn't have to do that; he *knew* from his experience and expertise that I no doubt had the condition. He also understood, because I had told him, that a year's worth of supplement iodine had not seemed to help much. Being a competent AK physician, he went through involved muscle-testing procedures to evaluate whether my metabolism was making use of the nutrients available in my bloodstream, and his thoroughness agreed with other personal information about me that my absorption of several nutrients, including calcium, was poor.

If the AK physician you approach explains the subject thoroughly, and at the same time explains that AK is primarily a tool helping him to evaluate your total body condition, and not some miracle cure-all process, then stick with him, or her; you've found a professional.

You may contact the ICAK to locate a member near you, if one exists, and to check your intended physician's standing within the only accredited organization in applied kinesiology:

International College of Applied Kinesiology,
P. O. Box 680547,
Park City,
Utah 84068.

Alternatively residents in Great Britain may contact the following address for information:

The British Touch for Health Association,
29 Bushey Close,
High Wycombe,
Bucks HP12 3HL.
Telephone: 0494 37409.

Finally, there are the considerations we must grant the medical establishment. You will not find traditional M.D.'s throwing any bouquets in the direction of applied kinesiology. Traditionally, the medical establishment resists change, and the history of medicine is story after story of a brilliant physician learning something new and struggling to overcome the built-in dogma. For example, incredible as it may seem, it took four hundred years for medical science to accept that nutrition could cure scurvy. However, when dealing with human health and lives, perhaps it's better to move slowly, despite the severe criticism received from observers with 20-20 hindsight. The premature acceptance of the drug thalidomide is a good example of what can happen when the medical establishment is less dogmatic and demanding. However, after having given the devil his due, we are of the opinion that the medical establishment needs to come off its high horse regarding applied kinesiology and begin to adopt the tried and true procedures.

John Diamond, M.D., began looking into AK procedures with a skeptical eye, but by being fair-minded he was able to learn the value of applied kinesiology and subsequently contribute considerably to AK lore. Diamond, a psychiatrist, wrote *Behavioural Kinesiology,* published by Harper and Row in 1979.

To illustrate what can be accomplished when medical doctors

are open-minded and willing to accept new ideas, we close this book with a review of Dr Diamond's work. He, too, came under the influence of the Goodheart genius, and aptly put the tenets of applied kinesiology to work in his psychiatric speciality in a unique, fascinating and apparently quite effective way.

Diamond's book opens with his views of 'energy level' and how a high level of energy signifies a state of health. He wrote: 'It appears that a generalized reduction of energy leads to energy imbalances in particular parts of the body. If we become aware of these energy imbalances when they first occur, we have a long grace period in which to correct them. We will then be practicing primary prevention.'

He distinguishes between 'primary' preventive medicine and 'secondary' preventive medicine. An example of the latter would be 'I've had a heart attack; prevent me from having another.'

Since psychiatry deals with the so-called psychosomatic influences (wherein our emotions cause physical symptoms), the experiences of Dr Diamond dovetailed with much of the information he learned from Dr Goodheart. Muscle-testing procedures, he determined, were ideal for treating his patients 'more completely than ever before. I was out of the narrow psychiatric framework and into what we may call a general preventive, energy-raising type of practice.' His conclusion supports what we have earlier stressed about the advantages of AK diagnosis on the hoof, so to speak, where the evaluations are on a living, breathing person.

After studying with Dr Goodheart, Dr Diamond said, 'For the first time, nutrition made sense to me.' The statement from the M.D. indicates that medical doctors not only fail to get a thorough education in nutrition while in medical school, but they are conditioned to sneer at nutritional precepts.

Dr Diamond used his own initiative and developed a brand of applied kinesiology called 'behavioral kinesiology (BK), an integration of psychiatry, psychosomatic medicine, kinesiology, preventive medicine and the humanities.' Much of his work centers around the thymus gland. In his book he calls the thymus a 'mysterious' gland and sketches some of the tragic history of medicine relative to the misconceptions about the thymus. For example, he points out that standard medical teaching still informs the medical doctors that the thymus has no function whatsoever in the adult. This is not true, he emphasizes: 'The evidence accumulated over the last twenty years on the thymus gland's role in immunology is so overwhelming that it is hard for me to believe that there is not some unconscious factor working to deny it the recognition due to it.'

Dr Diamond explains that the 'delusion' of the 'useless' thymus derived from autopsies that indicated the thymus was shriveled and atrophied, therefore not functional. This led to the erroneous conclusion that it was functionally useless in adults, when the truth is, the thymus responds to acute stress, and such hard work is known to have caused it to shrivel in twenty-four hours. Conversely, enlarged thymus glands in 'crib death' autopsies led to the equally erroneous conclusion that came to be labeled 'status thymicolymphaticus,' a dreadful disease that never really existed.

When I was a youth and under the wonderful influence of high-school education, I recall being taught that we humans evolved so that we no longer needed certain body parts, and this was 'established scientific fact.' The most common example given was the appendix. This intestinal appendage, we eager youngsters were told, served as a drain trap, so to speak, when we humans walked on all fours; but now that we walk upright, it is useless. Today it is known that both the appendix and the tonsils serve useful purposes as conduits from the lymph system into the blood.

Dr Diamond's BK thrust is expressed clearly in the book's subtitle: 'How to Activate Your Thymus and Increase Your Life Energy.' He devotes the bulk of the text to the importance of good posture, good food and good music. The 'good music' part is worthy of additional comment as it serves to further impress us with the evaluation abilities of applied kinesiology.

Dr Diamond cites the advanced ages attained by many famous classical musicians and suggests that the 'good music' played a role in their longevity. For example, Pablo Casals has reached 96, Rudolph Ganz 95, Leopold Stokowki 95, David Mannes 93, Ettore Panizza and Paul Paray 92, Arturo Toscanini 89, and so forth.

Dr Diamond then suggests the music played a role in their 'energy levels,' which enhanced their health and longevity. He discusses 'inner music' within our bodies and then tells of his experiments muscle-testing people while they were under the influence of various kinds of music.

For those conservative folk who wish to remark on it, yes, Dr Diamond did discover that some music was deleterious to energy level and therefore to health, and, yes, the worst music was, indeed, hard rock.

Applied kinesiology is in its infancy, and there will be many more innovative researchers like John Diamond coming under the influence of this intriguing, and helpful, form of medicine. While it is still struggling for recognition, you may employ added caution when seeking a qualified and competent AK physician. Armed with this book, it is our hope that you can now make excellent judgment.

Index